AF725287

Caregiver Logbook & Daily Health Tracker

A 90-Day Caregiver Logbook. A Complete Patient Care Journal for Medication Tracking, Doctor Visits, Symptoms, Mood & Wellness Monitoring | Essential Organizer for Family Caregivers

Daniel Harper

Table of Contents

Introduction

Caring for another person is one of the most meaningful and challenging responsibilities anyone can take on.

Whether you are caring for an aging parent, a spouse, a family member, or someone with a medical condition, your role as a caregiver requires patience, attention, and compassion every single day.

At times, caregiving can also feel overwhelming.

There are medications to remember, appointments to schedule, symptoms to monitor, and daily care tasks to manage. On top of that, caregivers often carry emotional and mental stress while trying to do their best for someone they deeply care about.

This **Caregiver Daily Logbook** was created to make that responsibility a little easier.

By keeping important information organized in one place, this logbook helps you track health details, medications, ,behaviour s, appointments, and daily care routines. Having a clear record can make it easier to notice changes in health, communicate with doctors, and provide better care over time.

Just as importantly, this book also encourages caregivers to take a moment to reflect on their own well-being. Caregivers often focus entirely on the person they are supporting, but your health and peace of mind matter too.

This logbook is not meant to add more work to your day. Instead, it is designed to be a simple tool that helps you stay organized, reduce stress, and feel more confident in the care you provide.

There is no perfect way to be a caregiver. Every situation is different, and every day brings new experiences.

But with patience, attention, and love, caregivers make an extraordinary difference in the lives of others.

This book is here to support you on that journey.

Section 1
Important Information

When caring for someone with medical needs, having important information organized in one place can save time and reduce stress. In an emergency or during a medical appointment, quick access to essential details can make communication with doctors, nurses, and caregivers much easier.

This section is designed to help you record key personal, medical, and contact information for the person in your care. You may also find it helpful to bring this logbook to doctor visits or hospital appointments so that healthcare professionals can quickly understand the patient's medical background.

Take a few minutes to fill out the following pages carefully. Update the information whenever there are changes to medications, doctors, or health conditions.

Keeping this information organized ensures that anyone assisting with care has access to accurate and up-to-date details.

Patient Information

Patient Name: ______________________________

Date of Birth: ______________________________

Age: ______________________________

Gender: ______________________________

Blood Type (if known): ______________________________

Home Address:

____

____

Primary Language: ______________________________

Emergency Contact Name: ______________________________

Relationship: ______________________________

Phone Number: ______________________________

Medical Conditions

Please list all current medical conditions or diagnoses.

1. ____________________
2. ____________________
3. ____________________
4. ____________________
5. ____________________

Additional Notes:

____

____

____

Allergies

List any known allergies, including medication, food, or environmental allergies.

1. ____________________
2. ____________________
3. ____________________
4. ____________________

Reaction Type (if known):

____

____

Primary Doctor Information

Doctor Name: ____________________

Clinic / Hospital Name: ____________________

Phone Number: ____________________

Address:

____

____

Email (if available): ___________________________

Specialist Doctors

Specialist Name: ___________________________

Specialty: ___________________________

Phone Number: ___________________________

Clinic / Hospital: ___________________________

Notes:

(Repeat this section if multiple specialists are involved.)

Pharmacy Information

Pharmacy Name: ___________________________

Phone Number: ___________________________

Address:

Preferred Pharmacist (if applicable): ___________________________

Insurance Information

Insurance Provider: ___________________________

Policy Number: ___________________________

Group Number: ___________________________

Customer Service Phone Number: ___________________________

Additional Notes:

Emergency Medical Information

In case of emergency, it is helpful for healthcare providers to know the following:

Current Medications:

Major Medical History:

Implants or Medical Devices (pacemaker, etc.):

Advance Directives / Living Will:
Yes / No

Location of Documents:

Caregiver Information

Primary Caregiver Name: ______________________________

Relationship to Patient: ______________________________

Phone Number: ______________________________

Secondary Caregiver Name: ______________________________

Phone Number: ______________________________

Important Notes

Use this space to write any additional information that may be helpful for medical professionals or other caregivers.

Section 2
Medication Tracker

Managing medications carefully is an important part of providing safe and effective care. Many individuals require multiple medications each day, often at different times. Keeping an accurate record helps ensure that medications are taken correctly and can also help doctors monitor treatment progress.

Use the following pages to record all medications given each day. You may also note any side effects, missed doses, or unusual reactions. This information can be very helpful during doctor visits or medical consultations.

If a medication routine changes, simply begin a new record on the next page.

Current Medication List

Before beginning daily tracking, it is helpful to list all current medications here.

Medication Name	Dosage	Frequency	Prescribing Doctor	Notes

Helpful Tip for Caregivers

It may be helpful to review medication records regularly and bring this logbook to doctor appointments. Accurate records help healthcare providers adjust medications safely and effectively.

Day: 1 Date:___________

Daily Medication Log

Use this table to record medications given each day.

Date	Medication Name	Dosage	Time Given	Given By	Side Effects / Notes

---

Missed or Delayed Medication Record

If a medication is missed or delayed, record it here.

Date	Medication	Scheduled Time	Reason Missed or Delayed	Action Taken

---

Medication Reaction or Side Effect Notes

Use this section to document any noticeable reactions or side effects after medications are taken.

Date: ______________________

Medication: ______________________

Observed Reaction / Side Effect:

Action Taken:

Doctor Notified: Yes / No

Day: 2 Date:___________

Daily Medication Log

Use this table to record medications given each day.

Date	Medication Name	Dosage	Time Given	Given By	Side Effects / Notes

---

Missed or Delayed Medication Record

If a medication is missed or delayed, record it here.

Date	Medication	Scheduled Time	Reason Missed or Delayed	Action Taken

---

Medication Reaction or Side Effect Notes

Use this section to document any noticeable reactions or side effects after medications are taken.

Date: ______________________

Medication: ______________________

Observed Reaction / Side Effect:

Action Taken:

Doctor Notified: Yes / No

Day: 3 Date:____________

Daily Medication Log

Use this table to record medications given each day.

Date	Medication Name	Dosage	Time Given	Given By	Side Effects / Notes

---

Missed or Delayed Medication Record

If a medication is missed or delayed, record it here.

Date	Medication	Scheduled Time	Reason Missed or Delayed	Action Taken

---

Medication Reaction or Side Effect Notes

Use this section to document any noticeable reactions or side effects after medications are taken.

Date: ______________________

Medication: ______________________

Observed Reaction / Side Effect:

Action Taken:

Doctor Notified: Yes / No

Day: 4 Date:___________

Daily Medication Log

Use this table to record medications given each day.

Date	Medication Name	Dosage	Time Given	Given By	Side Effects / Notes

---

Missed or Delayed Medication Record

If a medication is missed or delayed, record it here.

Date	Medication	Scheduled Time	Reason Missed or Delayed	Action Taken

---

Medication Reaction or Side Effect Notes

Use this section to document any noticeable reactions or side effects after medications are taken.

Date: ______________________

Medication: ______________________

Observed Reaction / Side Effect:

Action Taken:

Doctor Notified: Yes / No

Day: 5 Date:____________

Daily Medication Log

Use this table to record medications given each day.

Date	Medication Name	Dosage	Time Given	Given By	Side Effects / Notes

---

Missed or Delayed Medication Record

If a medication is missed or delayed, record it here.

Date	Medication	Scheduled Time	Reason Missed or Delayed	Action Taken

---

Medication Reaction or Side Effect Notes

Use this section to document any noticeable reactions or side effects after medications are taken.

Date: ______________________

Medication: ______________________

Observed Reaction / Side Effect:

Action Taken:

Doctor Notified: Yes / No

Day: 6 Date:___________

Daily Medication Log

Use this table to record medications given each day.

Date	Medication Name	Dosage	Time Given	Given By	Side Effects / Notes

---

Missed or Delayed Medication Record

If a medication is missed or delayed, record it here.

Date	Medication	Scheduled Time	Reason Missed or Delayed	Action Taken

---

Medication Reaction or Side Effect Notes

Use this section to document any noticeable reactions or side effects after medications are taken.

Date: ____________________

Medication: ____________________

Observed Reaction / Side Effect:

Action Taken:

Doctor Notified: Yes / No

Day: 7 Date:___________

Daily Medication Log

Use this table to record medications given each day.

Date	Medication Name	Dosage	Time Given	Given By	Side Effects / Notes

---

Missed or Delayed Medication Record

If a medication is missed or delayed, record it here.

Date	Medication	Scheduled Time	Reason Missed or Delayed	Action Taken

---

Medication Reaction or Side Effect Notes

Use this section to document any noticeable reactions or side effects after medications are taken.

Date: ____________________

Medication: ____________________

Observed Reaction / Side Effect:

Action Taken:

Doctor Notified: Yes / No

Day: 8 Date:___________

Daily Medication Log

Use this table to record medications given each day.

Date	Medication Name	Dosage	Time Given	Given By	Side Effects / Notes

---

Missed or Delayed Medication Record

If a medication is missed or delayed, record it here.

Date	Medication	Scheduled Time	Reason Missed or Delayed	Action Taken

---

Medication Reaction or Side Effect Notes

Use this section to document any noticeable reactions or side effects after medications are taken.

Date: ______________________

Medication: ______________________

Observed Reaction / Side Effect:

Action Taken:

Doctor Notified: Yes / No

Day: 9 Date:____________

Daily Medication Log

Use this table to record medications given each day.

Date	Medication Name	Dosage	Time Given	Given By	Side Effects / Notes

---

Missed or Delayed Medication Record

If a medication is missed or delayed, record it here.

Date	Medication	Scheduled Time	Reason Missed or Delayed	Action Taken

---

Medication Reaction or Side Effect Notes

Use this section to document any noticeable reactions or side effects after medications are taken.

Date: ______________________

Medication: ______________________

Observed Reaction / Side Effect:

Action Taken:

Doctor Notified: Yes / No

Day: 10 Date:____________

Daily Medication Log

Use this table to record medications given each day.

Date	Medication Name	Dosage	Time Given	Given By	Side Effects / Notes

---

Missed or Delayed Medication Record

If a medication is missed or delayed, record it here.

Date	Medication	Scheduled Time	Reason Missed or Delayed	Action Taken

---

Medication Reaction or Side Effect Notes

Use this section to document any noticeable reactions or side effects after medications are taken.

Date: ______________________

Medication: ______________________

Observed Reaction / Side Effect:

Action Taken:

Doctor Notified: Yes / No

Day: 11 **Date:____________**

Daily Medication Log

Use this table to record medications given each day.

Date	Medication Name	Dosage	Time Given	Given By	Side Effects / Notes

---

Missed or Delayed Medication Record

If a medication is missed or delayed, record it here.

Date	Medication	Scheduled Time	Reason Missed or Delayed	Action Taken

---

Medication Reaction or Side Effect Notes

Use this section to document any noticeable reactions or side effects after medications are taken.

Date: ______________________

Medication: ______________________

Observed Reaction / Side Effect:

Action Taken:

Doctor Notified: Yes / No

Day: 12 **Date:___________**

Daily Medication Log

Use this table to record medications given each day.

Date	Medication Name	Dosage	Time Given	Given By	Side Effects / Notes

---

Missed or Delayed Medication Record

If a medication is missed or delayed, record it here.

Date	Medication	Scheduled Time	Reason Missed or Delayed	Action Taken

---

Medication Reaction or Side Effect Notes

Use this section to document any noticeable reactions or side effects after medications are taken.

Date: ____________________

Medication: ____________________

Observed Reaction / Side Effect:

Action Taken:

Doctor Notified: Yes / No

Day: 13 Date:___________

Daily Medication Log

Use this table to record medications given each day.

Date	Medication Name	Dosage	Time Given	Given By	Side Effects / Notes

---

Missed or Delayed Medication Record

If a medication is missed or delayed, record it here.

Date	Medication	Scheduled Time	Reason Missed or Delayed	Action Taken

---

Medication Reaction or Side Effect Notes

Use this section to document any noticeable reactions or side effects after medications are taken.

Date: ____________________

Medication: ____________________

Observed Reaction / Side Effect:

Action Taken:

Doctor Notified: Yes / No

Day: 14 Date:___________

Daily Medication Log

Use this table to record medications given each day.

Date	Medication Name	Dosage	Time Given	Given By	Side Effects / Notes

---

Missed or Delayed Medication Record

If a medication is missed or delayed, record it here.

Date	Medication	Scheduled Time	Reason Missed or Delayed	Action Taken

---

Medication Reaction or Side Effect Notes

Use this section to document any noticeable reactions or side effects after medications are taken.

Date: ____________________

Medication: ____________________

Observed Reaction / Side Effect:

Action Taken:

Doctor Notified: Yes / No

Day: 15 Date:___________

Daily Medication Log

Use this table to record medications given each day.

Date	Medication Name	Dosage	Time Given	Given By	Side Effects / Notes

---

Missed or Delayed Medication Record

If a medication is missed or delayed, record it here.

Date	Medication	Scheduled Time	Reason Missed or Delayed	Action Taken

---

Medication Reaction or Side Effect Notes

Use this section to document any noticeable reactions or side effects after medications are taken.

Date: ____________________

Medication: ____________________

Observed Reaction / Side Effect:

Action Taken:

Doctor Notified: Yes / No

Day: 16 Date:___________

Daily Medication Log

Use this table to record medications given each day.

Date	Medication Name	Dosage	Time Given	Given By	Side Effects / Notes

---

Missed or Delayed Medication Record

If a medication is missed or delayed, record it here.

Date	Medication	Scheduled Time	Reason Missed or Delayed	Action Taken

---

Medication Reaction or Side Effect Notes

Use this section to document any noticeable reactions or side effects after medications are taken.

Date: ____________________

Medication: ____________________

Observed Reaction / Side Effect:

Action Taken:

Doctor Notified: Yes / No

Day: 17 **Date:____________**

Daily Medication Log

Use this table to record medications given each day.

Date	Medication Name	Dosage	Time Given	Given By	Side Effects / Notes

---

Missed or Delayed Medication Record

If a medication is missed or delayed, record it here.

Date	Medication	Scheduled Time	Reason Missed or Delayed	Action Taken

---

Medication Reaction or Side Effect Notes

Use this section to document any noticeable reactions or side effects after medications are taken.

Date: ______________________

Medication: ______________________

Observed Reaction / Side Effect:

Action Taken:

Doctor Notified: Yes / No

Day: 18 **Date:___________**

Daily Medication Log

Use this table to record medications given each day.

Date	Medication Name	Dosage	Time Given	Given By	Side Effects / Notes

---

Missed or Delayed Medication Record

If a medication is missed or delayed, record it here.

Date	Medication	Scheduled Time	Reason Missed or Delayed	Action Taken

---

Medication Reaction or Side Effect Notes

Use this section to document any noticeable reactions or side effects after medications are taken.

Date: ____________________

Medication: ____________________

Observed Reaction / Side Effect:

Action Taken:

Doctor Notified: Yes / No

Day: 19 **Date:____________**

Daily Medication Log

Use this table to record medications given each day.

Date	Medication Name	Dosage	Time Given	Given By	Side Effects / Notes

---

Missed or Delayed Medication Record

If a medication is missed or delayed, record it here.

Date	Medication	Scheduled Time	Reason Missed or Delayed	Action Taken

---

Medication Reaction or Side Effect Notes

Use this section to document any noticeable reactions or side effects after medications are taken.

Date: ____________________

Medication: ____________________

Observed Reaction / Side Effect:

Action Taken:

Doctor Notified: Yes / No

Day: 20 **Date:___________**

Daily Medication Log

Use this table to record medications given each day.

Date	Medication Name	Dosage	Time Given	Given By	Side Effects / Notes

---

Missed or Delayed Medication Record

If a medication is missed or delayed, record it here.

Date	Medication	Scheduled Time	Reason Missed or Delayed	Action Taken

---

Medication Reaction or Side Effect Notes

Use this section to document any noticeable reactions or side effects after medications are taken.

Date: ______________________

Medication: ______________________

Observed Reaction / Side Effect:

Action Taken:

Doctor Notified: Yes / No

Day: 21 **Date:____________**

Daily Medication Log

Use this table to record medications given each day.

Date	Medication Name	Dosage	Time Given	Given By	Side Effects / Notes

---

Missed or Delayed Medication Record

If a medication is missed or delayed, record it here.

Date	Medication	Scheduled Time	Reason Missed or Delayed	Action Taken

---

Medication Reaction or Side Effect Notes

Use this section to document any noticeable reactions or side effects after medications are taken.

Date: ______________________

Medication: ______________________

Observed Reaction / Side Effect:

Action Taken:

Doctor Notified: Yes / No

Day: 22 **Date:____________**

Daily Medication Log

Use this table to record medications given each day.

Date	Medication Name	Dosage	Time Given	Given By	Side Effects / Notes

---

Missed or Delayed Medication Record

If a medication is missed or delayed, record it here.

Date	Medication	Scheduled Time	Reason Missed or Delayed	Action Taken

---

Medication Reaction or Side Effect Notes

Use this section to document any noticeable reactions or side effects after medications are taken.

Date: ______________________

Medication: ______________________

Observed Reaction / Side Effect:

Action Taken:

Doctor Notified: Yes / No

Day: 23 Date:___________

Daily Medication Log

Use this table to record medications given each day.

Date	Medication Name	Dosage	Time Given	Given By	Side Effects / Notes

---

Missed or Delayed Medication Record

If a medication is missed or delayed, record it here.

Date	Medication	Scheduled Time	Reason Missed or Delayed	Action Taken

---

Medication Reaction or Side Effect Notes

Use this section to document any noticeable reactions or side effects after medications are taken.

Date: ______________________

Medication: ______________________

Observed Reaction / Side Effect:

Action Taken:

Doctor Notified: Yes / No

Day: 24 **Date:___________**

Daily Medication Log

Use this table to record medications given each day.

Date	Medication Name	Dosage	Time Given	Given By	Side Effects / Notes

---

Missed or Delayed Medication Record

If a medication is missed or delayed, record it here.

Date	Medication	Scheduled Time	Reason Missed or Delayed	Action Taken

---

Medication Reaction or Side Effect Notes

Use this section to document any noticeable reactions or side effects after medications are taken.

Date: ______________________

Medication: ______________________

Observed Reaction / Side Effect:

Action Taken:

Doctor Notified: Yes / No

Day: 25 **Date:___________**

Daily Medication Log

Use this table to record medications given each day.

Date	Medication Name	Dosage	Time Given	Given By	Side Effects / Notes

---

Missed or Delayed Medication Record

If a medication is missed or delayed, record it here.

Date	Medication	Scheduled Time	Reason Missed or Delayed	Action Taken

---

Medication Reaction or Side Effect Notes

Use this section to document any noticeable reactions or side effects after medications are taken.

Date: ______________________

Medication: ______________________

Observed Reaction / Side Effect:

Action Taken:

Doctor Notified: Yes / No

Day: 26 Date:___________

Daily Medication Log

Use this table to record medications given each day.

Date	Medication Name	Dosage	Time Given	Given By	Side Effects / Notes

---

Missed or Delayed Medication Record

If a medication is missed or delayed, record it here.

Date	Medication	Scheduled Time	Reason Missed or Delayed	Action Taken

---

Medication Reaction or Side Effect Notes

Use this section to document any noticeable reactions or side effects after medications are taken.

Date: ______________________

Medication: ______________________

Observed Reaction / Side Effect:

Action Taken:

Doctor Notified: Yes / No

Day: 27 **Date:___________**

Daily Medication Log

Use this table to record medications given each day.

Date	Medication Name	Dosage	Time Given	Given By	Side Effects / Notes

---

Missed or Delayed Medication Record

If a medication is missed or delayed, record it here.

Date	Medication	Scheduled Time	Reason Missed or Delayed	Action Taken

---

Medication Reaction or Side Effect Notes

Use this section to document any noticeable reactions or side effects after medications are taken.

Date: ______________________

Medication: ______________________

Observed Reaction / Side Effect:

Action Taken:

Doctor Notified: Yes / No

Day: 28

Daily Medication Log

Use this table to record medications given each day.

Date	Medication Name	Dosage	Time Given	Given By	Side Effects / Notes

---

Missed or Delayed Medication Record

If a medication is missed or delayed, record it here.

Date	Medication	Scheduled Time	Reason Missed or Delayed	Action Taken

---

Medication Reaction or Side Effect Notes

Use this section to document any noticeable reactions or side effects after medications are taken.

Date: ______________________

Medication: ______________________

Observed Reaction / Side Effect:

Action Taken:

Doctor Notified: Yes / No

Day: 29 **Date:____________**

Daily Medication Log

Use this table to record medications given each day.

Date	Medication Name	Dosage	Time Given	Given By	Side Effects / Notes

---

Missed or Delayed Medication Record

If a medication is missed or delayed, record it here.

Date	Medication	Scheduled Time	Reason Missed or Delayed	Action Taken

---

Medication Reaction or Side Effect Notes

Use this section to document any noticeable reactions or side effects after medications are taken.

Date: ______________________

Medication: ______________________

Observed Reaction / Side Effect:

Action Taken:

Doctor Notified: Yes / No

Day: 30 **Date:___________**

Daily Medication Log

Use this table to record medications given each day.

Date	Medication Name	Dosage	Time Given	Given By	Side Effects / Notes

---

Missed or Delayed Medication Record

If a medication is missed or delayed, record it here.

Date	Medication	Scheduled Time	Reason Missed or Delayed	Action Taken

---

Medication Reaction or Side Effect Notes

Use this section to document any noticeable reactions or side effects after medications are taken.

Date: ____________________

Medication: ____________________

Observed Reaction / Side Effect:

Action Taken:

Doctor Notified: Yes / No

Day: 31 **Date:___________**

Daily Medication Log

Use this table to record medications given each day.

Date	Medication Name	Dosage	Time Given	Given By	Side Effects / Notes

---

Missed or Delayed Medication Record

If a medication is missed or delayed, record it here.

Date	Medication	Scheduled Time	Reason Missed or Delayed	Action Taken

---

Medication Reaction or Side Effect Notes

Use this section to document any noticeable reactions or side effects after medications are taken.

Date: ____________________

Medication: ____________________

Observed Reaction / Side Effect:

Action Taken:

Doctor Notified: Yes / No

Day: 32 Date:___________

Daily Medication Log

Use this table to record medications given each day.

Date	Medication Name	Dosage	Time Given	Given By	Side Effects / Notes

---

Missed or Delayed Medication Record

If a medication is missed or delayed, record it here.

Date	Medication	Scheduled Time	Reason Missed or Delayed	Action Taken

---

Medication Reaction or Side Effect Notes

Use this section to document any noticeable reactions or side effects after medications are taken.

Date: ____________________

Medication: ____________________

Observed Reaction / Side Effect:

Action Taken:

Doctor Notified: Yes / No

Day: 33

Daily Medication Log

Use this table to record medications given each day.

Date	Medication Name	Dosage	Time Given	Given By	Side Effects / Notes

---

Missed or Delayed Medication Record

If a medication is missed or delayed, record it here.

Date	Medication	Scheduled Time	Reason Missed or Delayed	Action Taken

---

Medication Reaction or Side Effect Notes

Use this section to document any noticeable reactions or side effects after medications are taken.

Date: ______________________

Medication: ______________________

Observed Reaction / Side Effect:

Action Taken:

Doctor Notified: Yes / No

Day: 34 **Date:___________**

Daily Medication Log

Use this table to record medications given each day.

Date	Medication Name	Dosage	Time Given	Given By	Side Effects / Notes

---

Missed or Delayed Medication Record

If a medication is missed or delayed, record it here.

Date	Medication	Scheduled Time	Reason Missed or Delayed	Action Taken

---

Medication Reaction or Side Effect Notes

Use this section to document any noticeable reactions or side effects after medications are taken.

Date: ______________________

Medication: ______________________

Observed Reaction / Side Effect:

Action Taken:

Doctor Notified: Yes / No

Day: 35 Date:___________

Daily Medication Log

Use this table to record medications given each day.

Date	Medication Name	Dosage	Time Given	Given By	Side Effects / Notes

---

Missed or Delayed Medication Record

If a medication is missed or delayed, record it here.

Date	Medication	Scheduled Time	Reason Missed or Delayed	Action Taken

---

Medication Reaction or Side Effect Notes

Use this section to document any noticeable reactions or side effects after medications are taken.

Date: ______________________

Medication: ______________________

Observed Reaction / Side Effect:

Action Taken:

Doctor Notified: Yes / No

Day: 36 **Date:___________**

Daily Medication Log

Use this table to record medications given each day.

Date	Medication Name	Dosage	Time Given	Given By	Side Effects / Notes

---

Missed or Delayed Medication Record

If a medication is missed or delayed, record it here.

Date	Medication	Scheduled Time	Reason Missed or Delayed	Action Taken

---

Medication Reaction or Side Effect Notes

Use this section to document any noticeable reactions or side effects after medications are taken.

Date: ____________________

Medication: ____________________

Observed Reaction / Side Effect:

Action Taken:

Doctor Notified: Yes / No

Day: 37 Date:____________

Daily Medication Log

Use this table to record medications given each day.

Date	Medication Name	Dosage	Time Given	Given By	Side Effects / Notes

---

Missed or Delayed Medication Record

If a medication is missed or delayed, record it here.

Date	Medication	Scheduled Time	Reason Missed or Delayed	Action Taken

---

Medication Reaction or Side Effect Notes

Use this section to document any noticeable reactions or side effects after medications are taken.

Date: ______________________

Medication: ______________________

Observed Reaction / Side Effect:

Action Taken:

Doctor Notified: Yes / No

Day: 38 Date:___________

Daily Medication Log

Use this table to record medications given each day.

Date	Medication Name	Dosage	Time Given	Given By	Side Effects / Notes

---

Missed or Delayed Medication Record

If a medication is missed or delayed, record it here.

Date	Medication	Scheduled Time	Reason Missed or Delayed	Action Taken

---

Medication Reaction or Side Effect Notes

Use this section to document any noticeable reactions or side effects after medications are taken.

Date: ____________________

Medication: ____________________

Observed Reaction / Side Effect:

Action Taken:

Doctor Notified: Yes / No

Day: 39 **Date:____________**

Daily Medication Log

Use this table to record medications given each day.

Date	Medication Name	Dosage	Time Given	Given By	Side Effects / Notes

---

Missed or Delayed Medication Record

If a medication is missed or delayed, record it here.

Date	Medication	Scheduled Time	Reason Missed or Delayed	Action Taken

---

Medication Reaction or Side Effect Notes

Use this section to document any noticeable reactions or side effects after medications are taken.

Date: ____________________

Medication: ____________________

Observed Reaction / Side Effect:

Action Taken:

Doctor Notified: Yes / No

Day: 40 **Date:____________**

Daily Medication Log

Use this table to record medications given each day.

Date	Medication Name	Dosage	Time Given	Given By	Side Effects / Notes

---

Missed or Delayed Medication Record

If a medication is missed or delayed, record it here.

Date	Medication	Scheduled Time	Reason Missed or Delayed	Action Taken

---

Medication Reaction or Side Effect Notes

Use this section to document any noticeable reactions or side effects after medications are taken.

Date: ______________________

Medication: ______________________

Observed Reaction / Side Effect:

Action Taken:

Doctor Notified: Yes / No

Day: 41 **Date:____________**

Daily Medication Log

Use this table to record medications given each day.

Date	Medication Name	Dosage	Time Given	Given By	Side Effects / Notes

---

Missed or Delayed Medication Record

If a medication is missed or delayed, record it here.

Date	Medication	Scheduled Time	Reason Missed or Delayed	Action Taken

---

Medication Reaction or Side Effect Notes

Use this section to document any noticeable reactions or side effects after medications are taken.

Date: ______________________

Medication: ______________________

Observed Reaction / Side Effect:

Action Taken:

Doctor Notified: Yes / No

Day: 42 **Date:___________**

Daily Medication Log

Use this table to record medications given each day.

Date	Medication Name	Dosage	Time Given	Given By	Side Effects / Notes

---

Missed or Delayed Medication Record

If a medication is missed or delayed, record it here.

Date	Medication	Scheduled Time	Reason Missed or Delayed	Action Taken

---

Medication Reaction or Side Effect Notes

Use this section to document any noticeable reactions or side effects after medications are taken.

Date: ____________________

Medication: ____________________

Observed Reaction / Side Effect:

Action Taken:

Doctor Notified: Yes / No

Day: 43 **Date:____________**

Daily Medication Log

Use this table to record medications given each day.

Date	Medication Name	Dosage	Time Given	Given By	Side Effects / Notes

Missed or Delayed Medication Record

If a medication is missed or delayed, record it here.

Date	Medication	Scheduled Time	Reason Missed or Delayed	Action Taken

Medication Reaction or Side Effect Notes

Use this section to document any noticeable reactions or side effects after medications are taken.

Date: ______________________

Medication: ______________________

Observed Reaction / Side Effect:

Action Taken:

Doctor Notified: Yes / No

Day: 44 Date:____________

Daily Medication Log

Use this table to record medications given each day.

Date	Medication Name	Dosage	Time Given	Given By	Side Effects / Notes

---

Missed or Delayed Medication Record

If a medication is missed or delayed, record it here.

Date	Medication	Scheduled Time	Reason Missed or Delayed	Action Taken

---

Medication Reaction or Side Effect Notes

Use this section to document any noticeable reactions or side effects after medications are taken.

Date: ______________________

Medication: ______________________

Observed Reaction / Side Effect:

Action Taken:

Doctor Notified: Yes / No

Day: 45 **Date:____________**

Daily Medication Log

Use this table to record medications given each day.

Date	Medication Name	Dosage	Time Given	Given By	Side Effects / Notes

---

Missed or Delayed Medication Record

If a medication is missed or delayed, record it here.

Date	Medication	Scheduled Time	Reason Missed or Delayed	Action Taken

---

Medication Reaction or Side Effect Notes

Use this section to document any noticeable reactions or side effects after medications are taken.

Date: ______________________

Medication: ______________________

Observed Reaction / Side Effect:

Action Taken:

Doctor Notified: Yes / No

Day: 46　　**Date:___________**

Daily Medication Log

Use this table to record medications given each day.

Date	Medication Name	Dosage	Time Given	Given By	Side Effects / Notes

---

Missed or Delayed Medication Record

If a medication is missed or delayed, record it here.

Date	Medication	Scheduled Time	Reason Missed or Delayed	Action Taken

---

Medication Reaction or Side Effect Notes

Use this section to document any noticeable reactions or side effects after medications are taken.

Date: ______________________

Medication: ______________________

Observed Reaction / Side Effect:

Action Taken:

Doctor Notified: Yes / No

Day: 47 **Date:___________**

Daily Medication Log

Use this table to record medications given each day.

Date	Medication Name	Dosage	Time Given	Given By	Side Effects / Notes

---

Missed or Delayed Medication Record

If a medication is missed or delayed, record it here.

Date	Medication	Scheduled Time	Reason Missed or Delayed	Action Taken

---

Medication Reaction or Side Effect Notes

Use this section to document any noticeable reactions or side effects after medications are taken.

Date: ______________________

Medication: ______________________

Observed Reaction / Side Effect:

Action Taken:

Doctor Notified: Yes / No

Day: 48 **Date:____________**

Daily Medication Log

Use this table to record medications given each day.

Date	Medication Name	Dosage	Time Given	Given By	Side Effects / Notes

Missed or Delayed Medication Record

If a medication is missed or delayed, record it here.

Date	Medication	Scheduled Time	Reason Missed or Delayed	Action Taken

Medication Reaction or Side Effect Notes

Use this section to document any noticeable reactions or side effects after medications are taken.

Date: ______________________

Medication: ______________________

Observed Reaction / Side Effect:

Action Taken:

Doctor Notified: Yes / No

Day: 49 **Date:____________**

Daily Medication Log

Use this table to record medications given each day.

Date	Medication Name	Dosage	Time Given	Given By	Side Effects / Notes

---

Missed or Delayed Medication Record

If a medication is missed or delayed, record it here.

Date	Medication	Scheduled Time	Reason Missed or Delayed	Action Taken

---

Medication Reaction or Side Effect Notes

Use this section to document any noticeable reactions or side effects after medications are taken.

Date: ______________________

Medication: ______________________

Observed Reaction / Side Effect:

Action Taken:

Doctor Notified: Yes / No

Day: 50 **Date:___________**

Daily Medication Log

Use this table to record medications given each day.

Date	Medication Name	Dosage	Time Given	Given By	Side Effects / Notes

---

Missed or Delayed Medication Record

If a medication is missed or delayed, record it here.

Date	Medication	Scheduled Time	Reason Missed or Delayed	Action Taken

---

Medication Reaction or Side Effect Notes

Use this section to document any noticeable reactions or side effects after medications are taken.

Date: ______________________

Medication: ______________________

Observed Reaction / Side Effect:

Action Taken:

Doctor Notified: Yes / No

Day: 51 **Date:___________**

Daily Medication Log

Use this table to record medications given each day.

Date	Medication Name	Dosage	Time Given	Given By	Side Effects / Notes

---

Missed or Delayed Medication Record

If a medication is missed or delayed, record it here.

Date	Medication	Scheduled Time	Reason Missed or Delayed	Action Taken

---

Medication Reaction or Side Effect Notes

Use this section to document any noticeable reactions or side effects after medications are taken.

Date: ____________________

Medication: ____________________

Observed Reaction / Side Effect:

Action Taken:

Doctor Notified: Yes / No

Day: 52 **Date:___________**

Daily Medication Log

Use this table to record medications given each day.

Date	Medication Name	Dosage	Time Given	Given By	Side Effects / Notes

---

Missed or Delayed Medication Record

If a medication is missed or delayed, record it here.

Date	Medication	Scheduled Time	Reason Missed or Delayed	Action Taken

---

Medication Reaction or Side Effect Notes

Use this section to document any noticeable reactions or side effects after medications are taken.

Date: ____________________

Medication: ____________________

Observed Reaction / Side Effect:

Action Taken:

Doctor Notified: Yes / No

Day: 53 **Date:____________**

Daily Medication Log

Use this table to record medications given each day.

Date	Medication Name	Dosage	Time Given	Given By	Side Effects / Notes

---

Missed or Delayed Medication Record

If a medication is missed or delayed, record it here.

Date	Medication	Scheduled Time	Reason Missed or Delayed	Action Taken

---

Medication Reaction or Side Effect Notes

Use this section to document any noticeable reactions or side effects after medications are taken.

Date: ______________________

Medication: ______________________

Observed Reaction / Side Effect:

Action Taken:

Doctor Notified: Yes / No

Day: 54 Date:___________

Daily Medication Log

Use this table to record medications given each day.

Date	Medication Name	Dosage	Time Given	Given By	Side Effects / Notes

---

Missed or Delayed Medication Record

If a medication is missed or delayed, record it here.

Date	Medication	Scheduled Time	Reason Missed or Delayed	Action Taken

---

Medication Reaction or Side Effect Notes

Use this section to document any noticeable reactions or side effects after medications are taken.

Date: ____________________

Medication: ____________________

Observed Reaction / Side Effect:

Action Taken:

Doctor Notified: Yes / No

Day: 55 Date:____________

Daily Medication Log

Use this table to record medications given each day.

Date	Medication Name	Dosage	Time Given	Given By	Side Effects / Notes

---

Missed or Delayed Medication Record

If a medication is missed or delayed, record it here.

Date	Medication	Scheduled Time	Reason Missed or Delayed	Action Taken

---

Medication Reaction or Side Effect Notes

Use this section to document any noticeable reactions or side effects after medications are taken.

Date: ______________________

Medication: ______________________

Observed Reaction / Side Effect:

Action Taken:

Doctor Notified: Yes / No

Day: 56 **Date:____________**

Daily Medication Log

Use this table to record medications given each day.

Date	Medication Name	Dosage	Time Given	Given By	Side Effects / Notes

---

Missed or Delayed Medication Record

If a medication is missed or delayed, record it here.

Date	Medication	Scheduled Time	Reason Missed or Delayed	Action Taken

---

Medication Reaction or Side Effect Notes

Use this section to document any noticeable reactions or side effects after medications are taken.

Date: ______________________

Medication: ______________________

Observed Reaction / Side Effect:

Action Taken:

Doctor Notified: Yes / No

Day: 57 Date:____________

Daily Medication Log

Use this table to record medications given each day.

Date	Medication Name	Dosage	Time Given	Given By	Side Effects / Notes

Missed or Delayed Medication Record

If a medication is missed or delayed, record it here.

Date	Medication	Scheduled Time	Reason Missed or Delayed	Action Taken

Medication Reaction or Side Effect Notes

Use this section to document any noticeable reactions or side effects after medications are taken.

Date: ______________________

Medication: ______________________

Observed Reaction / Side Effect:

Action Taken:

Doctor Notified: Yes / No

Day: 58 **Date:____________**

Daily Medication Log

Use this table to record medications given each day.

Date	Medication Name	Dosage	Time Given	Given By	Side Effects / Notes

---

Missed or Delayed Medication Record

If a medication is missed or delayed, record it here.

Date	Medication	Scheduled Time	Reason Missed or Delayed	Action Taken

---

Medication Reaction or Side Effect Notes

Use this section to document any noticeable reactions or side effects after medications are taken.

Date: ______________________

Medication: ______________________

Observed Reaction / Side Effect:

Action Taken:

Doctor Notified: Yes / No

Day: 59 **Date:____________**

Daily Medication Log

Use this table to record medications given each day.

Date	Medication Name	Dosage	Time Given	Given By	Side Effects / Notes

---

Missed or Delayed Medication Record

If a medication is missed or delayed, record it here.

Date	Medication	Scheduled Time	Reason Missed or Delayed	Action Taken

---

Medication Reaction or Side Effect Notes

Use this section to document any noticeable reactions or side effects after medications are taken.

Date: ______________________

Medication: ______________________

Observed Reaction / Side Effect:

Action Taken:

Doctor Notified: Yes / No

Day: 60 **Date:___________**

Daily Medication Log

Use this table to record medications given each day.

Date	Medication Name	Dosage	Time Given	Given By	Side Effects / Notes

---

Missed or Delayed Medication Record

If a medication is missed or delayed, record it here.

Date	Medication	Scheduled Time	Reason Missed or Delayed	Action Taken

---

Medication Reaction or Side Effect Notes

Use this section to document any noticeable reactions or side effects after medications are taken.

Date: ______________________

Medication: ______________________

Observed Reaction / Side Effect:

Action Taken:

Doctor Notified: Yes / No

Day: 61 **Date:___________**

Daily Medication Log

Use this table to record medications given each day.

Date	Medication Name	Dosage	Time Given	Given By	Side Effects / Notes

Missed or Delayed Medication Record

If a medication is missed or delayed, record it here.

Date	Medication	Scheduled Time	Reason Missed or Delayed	Action Taken

Medication Reaction or Side Effect Notes

Use this section to document any noticeable reactions or side effects after medications are taken.

Date: ______________________

Medication: ______________________

Observed Reaction / Side Effect:

Action Taken:

Doctor Notified: Yes / No

Day: 62 **Date:____________**

Daily Medication Log

Use this table to record medications given each day.

Date	Medication Name	Dosage	Time Given	Given By	Side Effects / Notes

---

Missed or Delayed Medication Record

If a medication is missed or delayed, record it here.

Date	Medication	Scheduled Time	Reason Missed or Delayed	Action Taken

---

Medication Reaction or Side Effect Notes

Use this section to document any noticeable reactions or side effects after medications are taken.

Date: ______________________

Medication: ______________________

Observed Reaction / Side Effect:

Action Taken:

Doctor Notified: Yes / No

Day: 63 **Date:___________**

Daily Medication Log

Use this table to record medications given each day.

Date	Medication Name	Dosage	Time Given	Given By	Side Effects / Notes

---

Missed or Delayed Medication Record

If a medication is missed or delayed, record it here.

Date	Medication	Scheduled Time	Reason Missed or Delayed	Action Taken

---

Medication Reaction or Side Effect Notes

Use this section to document any noticeable reactions or side effects after medications are taken.

Date: ______________________

Medication: ______________________

Observed Reaction / Side Effect:

Action Taken:

Doctor Notified: Yes / No

Day: 64 **Date:___________**

Daily Medication Log

Use this table to record medications given each day.

Date	Medication Name	Dosage	Time Given	Given By	Side Effects / Notes

---

Missed or Delayed Medication Record

If a medication is missed or delayed, record it here.

Date	Medication	Scheduled Time	Reason Missed or Delayed	Action Taken

---

Medication Reaction or Side Effect Notes

Use this section to document any noticeable reactions or side effects after medications are taken.

Date: ____________________

Medication: ____________________

Observed Reaction / Side Effect:

Action Taken:

Doctor Notified: Yes / No

Day: 65 Date:____________

Daily Medication Log

Use this table to record medications given each day.

Date	Medication Name	Dosage	Time Given	Given By	Side Effects / Notes

---

Missed or Delayed Medication Record

If a medication is missed or delayed, record it here.

Date	Medication	Scheduled Time	Reason Missed or Delayed	Action Taken

---

Medication Reaction or Side Effect Notes

Use this section to document any noticeable reactions or side effects after medications are taken.

Date: ______________________

Medication: ______________________

Observed Reaction / Side Effect:

Action Taken:

Doctor Notified: Yes / No

Day: 66 **Date:____________**

Daily Medication Log

Use this table to record medications given each day.

Date	Medication Name	Dosage	Time Given	Given By	Side Effects / Notes

---

Missed or Delayed Medication Record

If a medication is missed or delayed, record it here.

Date	Medication	Scheduled Time	Reason Missed or Delayed	Action Taken

---

Medication Reaction or Side Effect Notes

Use this section to document any noticeable reactions or side effects after medications are taken.

Date: ______________________

Medication: ______________________

Observed Reaction / Side Effect:

Action Taken:

Doctor Notified: Yes / No

Day: 67 Date:___________

Daily Medication Log

Use this table to record medications given each day.

Date	Medication Name	Dosage	Time Given	Given By	Side Effects / Notes

---

Missed or Delayed Medication Record

If a medication is missed or delayed, record it here.

Date	Medication	Scheduled Time	Reason Missed or Delayed	Action Taken

---

Medication Reaction or Side Effect Notes

Use this section to document any noticeable reactions or side effects after medications are taken.

Date: ______________________

Medication: ______________________

Observed Reaction / Side Effect:

Action Taken:

Doctor Notified: Yes / No

Day: 68 **Date:____________**

Daily Medication Log

Use this table to record medications given each day.

Date	Medication Name	Dosage	Time Given	Given By	Side Effects / Notes

---

Missed or Delayed Medication Record

If a medication is missed or delayed, record it here.

Date	Medication	Scheduled Time	Reason Missed or Delayed	Action Taken

---

Medication Reaction or Side Effect Notes

Use this section to document any noticeable reactions or side effects after medications are taken.

Date: ______________________

Medication: ______________________

Observed Reaction / Side Effect:

Action Taken:

Doctor Notified: Yes / No

Day: 69 **Date:___________**

Daily Medication Log

Use this table to record medications given each day.

Date	Medication Name	Dosage	Time Given	Given By	Side Effects / Notes

---

Missed or Delayed Medication Record

If a medication is missed or delayed, record it here.

Date	Medication	Scheduled Time	Reason Missed or Delayed	Action Taken

---

Medication Reaction or Side Effect Notes

Use this section to document any noticeable reactions or side effects after medications are taken.

Date: ____________________

Medication: ____________________

Observed Reaction / Side Effect:

Action Taken:

Doctor Notified: Yes / No

Day: 70 **Date:____________**

Daily Medication Log

Use this table to record medications given each day.

Date	Medication Name	Dosage	Time Given	Given By	Side Effects / Notes

---

Missed or Delayed Medication Record

If a medication is missed or delayed, record it here.

Date	Medication	Scheduled Time	Reason Missed or Delayed	Action Taken

---

Medication Reaction or Side Effect Notes

Use this section to document any noticeable reactions or side effects after medications are taken.

Date: ______________________

Medication: ______________________

Observed Reaction / Side Effect:

Action Taken:

Doctor Notified: Yes / No

Day: 71 Date:___________

Daily Medication Log

Use this table to record medications given each day.

Date	Medication Name	Dosage	Time Given	Given By	Side Effects / Notes

---

Missed or Delayed Medication Record

If a medication is missed or delayed, record it here.

Date	Medication	Scheduled Time	Reason Missed or Delayed	Action Taken

---

Medication Reaction or Side Effect Notes

Use this section to document any noticeable reactions or side effects after medications are taken.

Date: ____________________

Medication: ____________________

Observed Reaction / Side Effect:

Action Taken:

Doctor Notified: Yes / No

Day: 72 Date:___________

Daily Medication Log

Use this table to record medications given each day.

Date	Medication Name	Dosage	Time Given	Given By	Side Effects / Notes

---

Missed or Delayed Medication Record

If a medication is missed or delayed, record it here.

Date	Medication	Scheduled Time	Reason Missed or Delayed	Action Taken

---

Medication Reaction or Side Effect Notes

Use this section to document any noticeable reactions or side effects after medications are taken.

Date: ____________________

Medication: ____________________

Observed Reaction / Side Effect:

Action Taken:

Doctor Notified: Yes / No

Day: 73 **Date:____________**

Daily Medication Log

Use this table to record medications given each day.

Date	Medication Name	Dosage	Time Given	Given By	Side Effects / Notes

---

Missed or Delayed Medication Record

If a medication is missed or delayed, record it here.

Date	Medication	Scheduled Time	Reason Missed or Delayed	Action Taken

---

Medication Reaction or Side Effect Notes

Use this section to document any noticeable reactions or side effects after medications are taken.

Date: ______________________

Medication: ______________________

Observed Reaction / Side Effect:

Action Taken:

Doctor Notified: Yes / No

Day: 74 **Date:___________**

Daily Medication Log

Use this table to record medications given each day.

Date	Medication Name	Dosage	Time Given	Given By	Side Effects / Notes

---

Missed or Delayed Medication Record

If a medication is missed or delayed, record it here.

Date	Medication	Scheduled Time	Reason Missed or Delayed	Action Taken

---

Medication Reaction or Side Effect Notes

Use this section to document any noticeable reactions or side effects after medications are taken.

Date: ______________________

Medication: ______________________

Observed Reaction / Side Effect:

Action Taken:

Doctor Notified: Yes / No

Day: 75 **Date:____________**

Daily Medication Log

Use this table to record medications given each day.

Date	Medication Name	Dosage	Time Given	Given By	Side Effects / Notes

Missed or Delayed Medication Record

If a medication is missed or delayed, record it here.

Date	Medication	Scheduled Time	Reason Missed or Delayed	Action Taken

Medication Reaction or Side Effect Notes

Use this section to document any noticeable reactions or side effects after medications are taken.

Date: ______________________

Medication: ______________________

Observed Reaction / Side Effect:

Action Taken:

Doctor Notified: Yes / No

Day: 76 **Date:___________**

Daily Medication Log

Use this table to record medications given each day.

Date	Medication Name	Dosage	Time Given	Given By	Side Effects / Notes

---

Missed or Delayed Medication Record

If a medication is missed or delayed, record it here.

Date	Medication	Scheduled Time	Reason Missed or Delayed	Action Taken

---

Medication Reaction or Side Effect Notes

Use this section to document any noticeable reactions or side effects after medications are taken.

Date: ______________________

Medication: ______________________

Observed Reaction / Side Effect:

Action Taken:

Doctor Notified: Yes / No

Day: 77 **Date:___________**

Daily Medication Log

Use this table to record medications given each day.

Date	Medication Name	Dosage	Time Given	Given By	Side Effects / Notes

---

Missed or Delayed Medication Record

If a medication is missed or delayed, record it here.

Date	Medication	Scheduled Time	Reason Missed or Delayed	Action Taken

---

Medication Reaction or Side Effect Notes

Use this section to document any noticeable reactions or side effects after medications are taken.

Date: ______________________

Medication: ______________________

Observed Reaction / Side Effect:

Action Taken:

Doctor Notified: Yes / No

Day: 78 **Date:___________**

Daily Medication Log

Use this table to record medications given each day.

Date	Medication Name	Dosage	Time Given	Given By	Side Effects / Notes

---

Missed or Delayed Medication Record

If a medication is missed or delayed, record it here.

Date	Medication	Scheduled Time	Reason Missed or Delayed	Action Taken

---

Medication Reaction or Side Effect Notes

Use this section to document any noticeable reactions or side effects after medications are taken.

Date: ______________________

Medication: ______________________

Observed Reaction / Side Effect:

Action Taken:

Doctor Notified: Yes / No

Day: 79 **Date:____________**

Daily Medication Log

Use this table to record medications given each day.

Date	Medication Name	Dosage	Time Given	Given By	Side Effects / Notes

---

Missed or Delayed Medication Record

If a medication is missed or delayed, record it here.

Date	Medication	Scheduled Time	Reason Missed or Delayed	Action Taken

---

Medication Reaction or Side Effect Notes

Use this section to document any noticeable reactions or side effects after medications are taken.

Date: ______________________

Medication: ______________________

Observed Reaction / Side Effect:

Action Taken:

Doctor Notified: Yes / No

Day: 80 **Date:____________**

Daily Medication Log

Use this table to record medications given each day.

Date	Medication Name	Dosage	Time Given	Given By	Side Effects / Notes

---

Missed or Delayed Medication Record

If a medication is missed or delayed, record it here.

Date	Medication	Scheduled Time	Reason Missed or Delayed	Action Taken

---

Medication Reaction or Side Effect Notes

Use this section to document any noticeable reactions or side effects after medications are taken.

Date: ______________________

Medication: ______________________

Observed Reaction / Side Effect:

Action Taken:

Doctor Notified: Yes / No

Day: 81 **Date:____________**

Daily Medication Log

Use this table to record medications given each day.

Date	Medication Name	Dosage	Time Given	Given By	Side Effects / Notes

---

Missed or Delayed Medication Record

If a medication is missed or delayed, record it here.

Date	Medication	Scheduled Time	Reason Missed or Delayed	Action Taken

---

Medication Reaction or Side Effect Notes

Use this section to document any noticeable reactions or side effects after medications are taken.

Date: ______________________

Medication: ______________________

Observed Reaction / Side Effect:

Action Taken:

Doctor Notified: Yes / No

Day: 82 **Date:___________**

Daily Medication Log

Use this table to record medications given each day.

Date	Medication Name	Dosage	Time Given	Given By	Side Effects / Notes

Missed or Delayed Medication Record

If a medication is missed or delayed, record it here.

Date	Medication	Scheduled Time	Reason Missed or Delayed	Action Taken

Medication Reaction or Side Effect Notes

Use this section to document any noticeable reactions or side effects after medications are taken.

Date: ______________________

Medication: ______________________

Observed Reaction / Side Effect:

Action Taken:

Doctor Notified: Yes / No

Day: 83 **Date:____________**

Daily Medication Log

Use this table to record medications given each day.

Date	Medication Name	Dosage	Time Given	Given By	Side Effects / Notes

Missed or Delayed Medication Record

If a medication is missed or delayed, record it here.

Date	Medication	Scheduled Time	Reason Missed or Delayed	Action Taken

Medication Reaction or Side Effect Notes

Use this section to document any noticeable reactions or side effects after medications are taken.

Date: ______________________

Medication: ______________________

Observed Reaction / Side Effect:

Action Taken:

Doctor Notified: Yes / No

Day: 84 Date:___________

Daily Medication Log

Use this table to record medications given each day.

Date	Medication Name	Dosage	Time Given	Given By	Side Effects / Notes

---

Missed or Delayed Medication Record

If a medication is missed or delayed, record it here.

Date	Medication	Scheduled Time	Reason Missed or Delayed	Action Taken

---

Medication Reaction or Side Effect Notes

Use this section to document any noticeable reactions or side effects after medications are taken.

Date: ______________________

Medication: ______________________

Observed Reaction / Side Effect:

Action Taken:

Doctor Notified: Yes / No

Day: 85 Date:____________

Daily Medication Log

Use this table to record medications given each day.

Date	Medication Name	Dosage	Time Given	Given By	Side Effects / Notes

---

Missed or Delayed Medication Record

If a medication is missed or delayed, record it here.

Date	Medication	Scheduled Time	Reason Missed or Delayed	Action Taken

---

Medication Reaction or Side Effect Notes

Use this section to document any noticeable reactions or side effects after medications are taken.

Date: ______________________

Medication: ______________________

Observed Reaction / Side Effect:

Action Taken:

Doctor Notified: Yes / No

Day: 86 **Date:___________**

Daily Medication Log

Use this table to record medications given each day.

Date	Medication Name	Dosage	Time Given	Given By	Side Effects / Notes

---

Missed or Delayed Medication Record

If a medication is missed or delayed, record it here.

Date	Medication	Scheduled Time	Reason Missed or Delayed	Action Taken

---

Medication Reaction or Side Effect Notes

Use this section to document any noticeable reactions or side effects after medications are taken.

Date: ______________________

Medication: ______________________

Observed Reaction / Side Effect:

Action Taken:

Doctor Notified: Yes / No

Day: 87 **Date:___________**

Daily Medication Log

Use this table to record medications given each day.

Date	Medication Name	Dosage	Time Given	Given By	Side Effects / Notes

---

Missed or Delayed Medication Record

If a medication is missed or delayed, record it here.

Date	Medication	Scheduled Time	Reason Missed or Delayed	Action Taken

---

Medication Reaction or Side Effect Notes

Use this section to document any noticeable reactions or side effects after medications are taken.

Date: ______________________

Medication: ______________________

Observed Reaction / Side Effect:

Action Taken:

Doctor Notified: Yes / No

Day: 88 Date:___________

Daily Medication Log

Use this table to record medications given each day.

Date	Medication Name	Dosage	Time Given	Given By	Side Effects / Notes

---

Missed or Delayed Medication Record

If a medication is missed or delayed, record it here.

Date	Medication	Scheduled Time	Reason Missed or Delayed	Action Taken

---

Medication Reaction or Side Effect Notes

Use this section to document any noticeable reactions or side effects after medications are taken.

Date: ______________________

Medication: ______________________

Observed Reaction / Side Effect:

Action Taken:

Doctor Notified: Yes / No

Day: 89 **Date:____________**

Daily Medication Log

Use this table to record medications given each day.

Date	Medication Name	Dosage	Time Given	Given By	Side Effects / Notes

---

Missed or Delayed Medication Record

If a medication is missed or delayed, record it here.

Date	Medication	Scheduled Time	Reason Missed or Delayed	Action Taken

---

Medication Reaction or Side Effect Notes

Use this section to document any noticeable reactions or side effects after medications are taken.

Date: ______________________

Medication: ______________________

Observed Reaction / Side Effect:

Action Taken:

Doctor Notified: Yes / No

Day: 90 **Date:____________**

Daily Medication Log

Use this table to record medications given each day.

Date	Medication Name	Dosage	Time Given	Given By	Side Effects / Notes

---

Missed or Delayed Medication Record

If a medication is missed or delayed, record it here.

Date	Medication	Scheduled Time	Reason Missed or Delayed	Action Taken

---

Medication Reaction or Side Effect Notes

Use this section to document any noticeable reactions or side effects after medications are taken.

Date: ______________________

Medication: ______________________

Observed Reaction / Side Effect:

Action Taken:

Doctor Notified: Yes / No

Section 3
Daily Health & Wellness Tracker

Monitoring daily health indicators can help caregivers notice important changes early. Small changes in sleep, appetite, mood, or physical comfort may signal developing health issues that require attention.

By recording these details each day, caregivers can provide doctors and healthcare professionals with useful information that may help guide treatment and care decisions.

This section allows you to track key health indicators on a daily basis. Try to record information at roughly the same time each day for consistency.

Remember that these records do not replace medical advice, but they can be extremely helpful when discussing health changes with a healthcare provider.

Daily Health & Wellness Log

Date: ________________ Day: 1

Health Indicator	Record / Observation
Blood Pressure	__________________
Blood Sugar (if applicable)	__________________
Temperature	__________________
Pulse / Heart Rate	__________________
Pain Level (1–10)	__________________
Hours of Sleep	__________________
Appetite	Poor / Normal / Good
Hydration	Low / Moderate / Good
Physical Activity	None / Light / Moderate
Mood	Calm / Happy / Irritable / Confused
Energy Level	Low / Medium / High

Daily Observations

Use this space to record any changes or important observations. Examples: confusion, dizziness, swelling, breathing difficulty, behavioural changes, or unusual symptoms.

Bowel Movement & Digestion Tracker

Digestive health is important for many patients, especially those with mobility or medication-related issues.

Bowel Movement	Yes / No
Digestive Discomfort	Yes / No
Notes	__________________

Sleep Quality Tracker

Sleep patterns often reveal important health signals.

Sleep Quality	**Excellent / Good / Fair / Poor**
Night Disturbances	Yes / No
Daytime Drowsiness	Yes / No

Notes:

Hydration & Nutrition Notes

Food and water intake are critical for recovery and health maintenance.

Meals Consumed Today:
Breakfast / Lunch / Dinner / Snacks

Hydration Level:
Low / Moderate / Good

Notes:

Warning Signs to Watch

Contact a healthcare professional if you notice:

- Sudden confusion or memory changes
- Difficulty breathing
- High fever
- Severe pain
- Persistent dizziness or weakness
- Unusual swelling

If symptoms appear serious, seek medical attention immediately.

Daily Health & Wellness Log

Date: ________________ Day: 2

Health Indicator	Record / Observation
Blood Pressure	________________
Blood Sugar (if applicable)	________________
Temperature	________________
Pulse / Heart Rate	________________
Pain Level (1–10)	________________
Hours of Sleep	________________
Appetite	Poor / Normal / Good
Hydration	Low / Moderate / Good
Physical Activity	None / Light / Moderate
Mood	Calm / Happy / Irritable / Confused
Energy Level	Low / Medium / High

Daily Observations

Use this space to record any changes or important observations. Examples: confusion, dizziness, swelling, breathing difficulty, behavioural changes, or unusual symptoms.

Bowel Movement & Digestion Tracker

Digestive health is important for many patients, especially those with mobility or medication-related issues.

Bowel Movement	Yes / No
Digestive Discomfort	Yes / No
Notes	________________

Sleep Quality Tracker

Sleep patterns often reveal important health signals.

Sleep Quality	**Excellent / Good / Fair / Poor**
Night Disturbances	Yes / No
Daytime Drowsiness	Yes / No

Notes:

Hydration & Nutrition Notes

Food and water intake are critical for recovery and health maintenance.

Meals Consumed Today:
Breakfast / Lunch / Dinner / Snacks

Hydration Level:
Low / Moderate / Good

Notes:

Warning Signs to Watch

Contact a healthcare professional if you notice:

- Sudden confusion or memory changes
- Difficulty breathing
- High fever
- Severe pain
- Persistent dizziness or weakness
- Unusual swelling

If symptoms appear serious, seek medical attention immediately.

Daily Health & Wellness Log

Date: ________________ Day: 3

Health Indicator	Record / Observation
Blood Pressure	__________________
Blood Sugar (if applicable)	__________________
Temperature	__________________
Pulse / Heart Rate	__________________
Pain Level (1–10)	__________________
Hours of Sleep	__________________
Appetite	Poor / Normal / Good
Hydration	Low / Moderate / Good
Physical Activity	None / Light / Moderate
Mood	Calm / Happy / Irritable / Confused
Energy Level	Low / Medium / High

Daily Observations

Use this space to record any changes or important observations. Examples: confusion, dizziness, swelling, breathing difficulty, behavioural changes, or unusual symptoms.

Bowel Movement & Digestion Tracker

Digestive health is important for many patients, especially those with mobility or medication-related issues.

Bowel Movement	Yes / No
Digestive Discomfort	Yes / No
Notes	__________________

Sleep Quality Tracker

Sleep patterns often reveal important health signals.

Sleep Quality	**Excellent / Good / Fair / Poor**
Night Disturbances	Yes / No
Daytime Drowsiness	Yes / No

Notes:

Hydration & Nutrition Notes

Food and water intake are critical for recovery and health maintenance.

Meals Consumed Today:
Breakfast / Lunch / Dinner / Snacks

Hydration Level:
Low / Moderate / Good

Notes:

Warning Signs to Watch

Contact a healthcare professional if you notice:

- Sudden confusion or memory changes
- Difficulty breathing
- High fever
- Severe pain
- Persistent dizziness or weakness
- Unusual swelling

If symptoms appear serious, seek medical attention immediately.

Daily Health & Wellness Log

Date: ________________ Day: 4

Health Indicator	Record / Observation
Blood Pressure	__________________
Blood Sugar (if applicable)	__________________
Temperature	__________________
Pulse / Heart Rate	__________________
Pain Level (1–10)	__________________
Hours of Sleep	__________________
Appetite	Poor / Normal / Good
Hydration	Low / Moderate / Good
Physical Activity	None / Light / Moderate
Mood	Calm / Happy / Irritable / Confused
Energy Level	Low / Medium / High

Daily Observations

Use this space to record any changes or important observations. Examples: confusion, dizziness, swelling, breathing difficulty, behavioural changes, or unusual symptoms.

Bowel Movement & Digestion Tracker

Digestive health is important for many patients, especially those with mobility or medication-related issues.

Bowel Movement	Yes / No
Digestive Discomfort	Yes / No
Notes	__________________

Sleep Quality Tracker

Sleep patterns often reveal important health signals.

Sleep Quality	**Excellent / Good / Fair / Poor**
Night Disturbances	Yes / No
Daytime Drowsiness	Yes / No

Notes:

Hydration & Nutrition Notes

Food and water intake are critical for recovery and health maintenance.

Meals Consumed Today:
Breakfast / Lunch / Dinner / Snacks

Hydration Level:
Low / Moderate / Good

Notes:

Warning Signs to Watch

Contact a healthcare professional if you notice:

- Sudden confusion or memory changes
- Difficulty breathing
- High fever
- Severe pain
- Persistent dizziness or weakness
- Unusual swelling

If symptoms appear serious, seek medical attention immediately.

Daily Health & Wellness Log

Date: _______________ Day: 5

Health Indicator	Record / Observation
Blood Pressure	_________________
Blood Sugar (if applicable)	_________________
Temperature	_________________
Pulse / Heart Rate	_________________
Pain Level (1–10)	_________________
Hours of Sleep	_________________
Appetite	Poor / Normal / Good
Hydration	Low / Moderate / Good
Physical Activity	None / Light / Moderate
Mood	Calm / Happy / Irritable / Confused
Energy Level	Low / Medium / High

Daily Observations

Use this space to record any changes or important observations. Examples: confusion, dizziness, swelling, breathing difficulty, behavioural changes, or unusual symptoms.

Bowel Movement & Digestion Tracker

Digestive health is important for many patients, especially those with mobility or medication-related issues.

Bowel Movement	Yes / No
Digestive Discomfort	Yes / No
Notes	_________________

Sleep Quality Tracker

Sleep patterns often reveal important health signals.

Sleep Quality	**Excellent / Good / Fair / Poor**
Night Disturbances	Yes / No
Daytime Drowsiness	Yes / No

Notes:

Hydration & Nutrition Notes

Food and water intake are critical for recovery and health maintenance.

Meals Consumed Today:
Breakfast / Lunch / Dinner / Snacks

Hydration Level:
Low / Moderate / Good

Notes:

Warning Signs to Watch

Contact a healthcare professional if you notice:

- Sudden confusion or memory changes
- Difficulty breathing
- High fever
- Severe pain
- Persistent dizziness or weakness
- Unusual swelling

If symptoms appear serious, seek medical attention immediately.

Daily Health & Wellness Log

Date: ________________ Day: 6

Health Indicator	Record / Observation
Blood Pressure	________________
Blood Sugar (if applicable)	________________
Temperature	________________
Pulse / Heart Rate	________________
Pain Level (1–10)	________________
Hours of Sleep	________________
Appetite	Poor / Normal / Good
Hydration	Low / Moderate / Good
Physical Activity	None / Light / Moderate
Mood	Calm / Happy / Irritable / Confused
Energy Level	Low / Medium / High

Daily Observations

Use this space to record any changes or important observations. Examples: confusion, dizziness, swelling, breathing difficulty, behavioural changes, or unusual symptoms.

Bowel Movement & Digestion Tracker

Digestive health is important for many patients, especially those with mobility or medication-related issues.

Bowel Movement	Yes / No
Digestive Discomfort	Yes / No
Notes	________________

Sleep Quality Tracker

Sleep patterns often reveal important health signals.

Sleep Quality	**Excellent / Good / Fair / Poor**
Night Disturbances	Yes / No
Daytime Drowsiness	Yes / No

Notes:

Hydration & Nutrition Notes

Food and water intake are critical for recovery and health maintenance.

Meals Consumed Today:
Breakfast / Lunch / Dinner / Snacks

Hydration Level:
Low / Moderate / Good

Notes:

Warning Signs to Watch

Contact a healthcare professional if you notice:

- Sudden confusion or memory changes
- Difficulty breathing
- High fever
- Severe pain
- Persistent dizziness or weakness
- Unusual swelling

If symptoms appear serious, seek medical attention immediately.

Daily Health & Wellness Log

Date: ________________ Day: 7

Health Indicator	Record / Observation
Blood Pressure	__________________
Blood Sugar (if applicable)	__________________
Temperature	__________________
Pulse / Heart Rate	__________________
Pain Level (1–10)	__________________
Hours of Sleep	__________________
Appetite	Poor / Normal / Good
Hydration	Low / Moderate / Good
Physical Activity	None / Light / Moderate
Mood	Calm / Happy / Irritable / Confused
Energy Level	Low / Medium / High

Daily Observations

Use this space to record any changes or important observations. Examples: confusion, dizziness, swelling, breathing difficulty, behavioural changes, or unusual symptoms.

Bowel Movement & Digestion Tracker

Digestive health is important for many patients, especially those with mobility or medication-related issues.

Bowel Movement	Yes / No
Digestive Discomfort	Yes / No
Notes	__________________

Sleep Quality Tracker

Sleep patterns often reveal important health signals.

Sleep Quality	**Excellent / Good / Fair / Poor**
Night Disturbances	Yes / No
Daytime Drowsiness	Yes / No

Notes:

Hydration & Nutrition Notes

Food and water intake are critical for recovery and health maintenance.

Meals Consumed Today:
Breakfast / Lunch / Dinner / Snacks

Hydration Level:
Low / Moderate / Good

Notes:

Warning Signs to Watch

Contact a healthcare professional if you notice:

- Sudden confusion or memory changes
- Difficulty breathing
- High fever
- Severe pain
- Persistent dizziness or weakness
- Unusual swelling

If symptoms appear serious, seek medical attention immediately.

Daily Health & Wellness Log

Date: ________________ Day: 8

Health Indicator	Record / Observation
Blood Pressure	__________________
Blood Sugar (if applicable)	__________________
Temperature	__________________
Pulse / Heart Rate	__________________
Pain Level (1–10)	__________________
Hours of Sleep	__________________
Appetite	Poor / Normal / Good
Hydration	Low / Moderate / Good
Physical Activity	None / Light / Moderate
Mood	Calm / Happy / Irritable / Confused
Energy Level	Low / Medium / High

Daily Observations

Use this space to record any changes or important observations. Examples: confusion, dizziness, swelling, breathing difficulty, behavioural changes, or unusual symptoms.

Bowel Movement & Digestion Tracker

Digestive health is important for many patients, especially those with mobility or medication-related issues.

Bowel Movement	Yes / No
Digestive Discomfort	Yes / No
Notes	__________________

Sleep Quality Tracker

Sleep patterns often reveal important health signals.

Sleep Quality	**Excellent / Good / Fair / Poor**
Night Disturbances	Yes / No
Daytime Drowsiness	Yes / No

Notes:

Hydration & Nutrition Notes

Food and water intake are critical for recovery and health maintenance.

Meals Consumed Today:
Breakfast / Lunch / Dinner / Snacks

Hydration Level:
Low / Moderate / Good

Notes:

Warning Signs to Watch

Contact a healthcare professional if you notice:

- Sudden confusion or memory changes
- Difficulty breathing
- High fever
- Severe pain
- Persistent dizziness or weakness
- Unusual swelling

If symptoms appear serious, seek medical attention immediately.

Daily Health & Wellness Log

Date: ________________ Day: 9

Health Indicator	Record / Observation
Blood Pressure	__________________
Blood Sugar (if applicable)	__________________
Temperature	__________________
Pulse / Heart Rate	__________________
Pain Level (1–10)	__________________
Hours of Sleep	__________________
Appetite	Poor / Normal / Good
Hydration	Low / Moderate / Good
Physical Activity	None / Light / Moderate
Mood	Calm / Happy / Irritable / Confused
Energy Level	Low / Medium / High

Daily Observations

Use this space to record any changes or important observations. Examples: confusion, dizziness, swelling, breathing difficulty, behavioural changes, or unusual symptoms.

Bowel Movement & Digestion Tracker

Digestive health is important for many patients, especially those with mobility or medication-related issues.

Bowel Movement	Yes / No
Digestive Discomfort	Yes / No
Notes	__________________

Sleep Quality Tracker

Sleep patterns often reveal important health signals.

Sleep Quality	**Excellent / Good / Fair / Poor**
Night Disturbances	Yes / No
Daytime Drowsiness	Yes / No

Notes:

Hydration & Nutrition Notes

Food and water intake are critical for recovery and health maintenance.

Meals Consumed Today:
Breakfast / Lunch / Dinner / Snacks

Hydration Level:
Low / Moderate / Good

Notes:

Warning Signs to Watch

Contact a healthcare professional if you notice:

- Sudden confusion or memory changes
- Difficulty breathing
- High fever
- Severe pain
- Persistent dizziness or weakness
- Unusual swelling

If symptoms appear serious, seek medical attention immediately.

Daily Health & Wellness Log

Date: ________________ Day: 10

Health Indicator	Record / Observation
Blood Pressure	________________
Blood Sugar (if applicable)	________________
Temperature	________________
Pulse / Heart Rate	________________
Pain Level (1–10)	________________
Hours of Sleep	________________
Appetite	Poor / Normal / Good
Hydration	Low / Moderate / Good
Physical Activity	None / Light / Moderate
Mood	Calm / Happy / Irritable / Confused
Energy Level	Low / Medium / High

Daily Observations

Use this space to record any changes or important observations. Examples: confusion, dizziness, swelling, breathing difficulty, behavioural changes, or unusual symptoms.

Bowel Movement & Digestion Tracker

Digestive health is important for many patients, especially those with mobility or medication-related issues.

Bowel Movement	Yes / No
Digestive Discomfort	Yes / No
Notes	________________

Sleep Quality Tracker

Sleep patterns often reveal important health signals.

Sleep Quality	**Excellent / Good / Fair / Poor**
Night Disturbances	Yes / No
Daytime Drowsiness	Yes / No

Notes:

Hydration & Nutrition Notes

Food and water intake are critical for recovery and health maintenance.

Meals Consumed Today:
Breakfast / Lunch / Dinner / Snacks

Hydration Level:
Low / Moderate / Good

Notes:

Warning Signs to Watch

Contact a healthcare professional if you notice:

- Sudden confusion or memory changes
- Difficulty breathing
- High fever
- Severe pain
- Persistent dizziness or weakness
- Unusual swelling

If symptoms appear serious, seek medical attention immediately.

Daily Health & Wellness Log

Date: ________________ Day: 11

Health Indicator	Record / Observation
Blood Pressure	________________
Blood Sugar (if applicable)	________________
Temperature	________________
Pulse / Heart Rate	________________
Pain Level (1–10)	________________
Hours of Sleep	________________
Appetite	Poor / Normal / Good
Hydration	Low / Moderate / Good
Physical Activity	None / Light / Moderate
Mood	Calm / Happy / Irritable / Confused
Energy Level	Low / Medium / High

Daily Observations

Use this space to record any changes or important observations. Examples: confusion, dizziness, swelling, breathing difficulty, behavioural changes, or unusual symptoms.

Bowel Movement & Digestion Tracker

Digestive health is important for many patients, especially those with mobility or medication-related issues.

Bowel Movement	Yes / No
Digestive Discomfort	Yes / No
Notes	________________

Sleep Quality Tracker

Sleep patterns often reveal important health signals.

Sleep Quality	Excellent / Good / Fair / Poor
Night Disturbances	Yes / No
Daytime Drowsiness	Yes / No

Notes:

Hydration & Nutrition Notes

Food and water intake are critical for recovery and health maintenance.

Meals Consumed Today:
Breakfast / Lunch / Dinner / Snacks

Hydration Level:
Low / Moderate / Good

Notes:

Warning Signs to Watch

Contact a healthcare professional if you notice:

- Sudden confusion or memory changes
- Difficulty breathing
- High fever
- Severe pain
- Persistent dizziness or weakness
- Unusual swelling

If symptoms appear serious, seek medical attention immediately.

Daily Health & Wellness Log

Date: ________________ Day: 12

Health Indicator	Record / Observation
Blood Pressure	__________________
Blood Sugar (if applicable)	__________________
Temperature	__________________
Pulse / Heart Rate	__________________
Pain Level (1–10)	__________________
Hours of Sleep	__________________
Appetite	Poor / Normal / Good
Hydration	Low / Moderate / Good
Physical Activity	None / Light / Moderate
Mood	Calm / Happy / Irritable / Confused
Energy Level	Low / Medium / High

Daily Observations

Use this space to record any changes or important observations. Examples: confusion, dizziness, swelling, breathing difficulty, behavioural changes, or unusual symptoms.

Bowel Movement & Digestion Tracker

Digestive health is important for many patients, especially those with mobility or medication-related issues.

Bowel Movement	Yes / No
Digestive Discomfort	Yes / No
Notes	__________________

Sleep Quality Tracker

Sleep patterns often reveal important health signals.

Sleep Quality	**Excellent / Good / Fair / Poor**
Night Disturbances	Yes / No
Daytime Drowsiness	Yes / No

Notes:

Hydration & Nutrition Notes

Food and water intake are critical for recovery and health maintenance.

Meals Consumed Today:
Breakfast / Lunch / Dinner / Snacks

Hydration Level:
Low / Moderate / Good

Notes:

Warning Signs to Watch

Contact a healthcare professional if you notice:

- Sudden confusion or memory changes
- Difficulty breathing
- High fever
- Severe pain
- Persistent dizziness or weakness
- Unusual swelling

If symptoms appear serious, seek medical attention immediately.

Daily Health & Wellness Log

Date: ________________ Day: 13

Health Indicator	Record / Observation
Blood Pressure	____________________
Blood Sugar (if applicable)	____________________
Temperature	____________________
Pulse / Heart Rate	____________________
Pain Level (1–10)	____________________
Hours of Sleep	____________________
Appetite	Poor / Normal / Good
Hydration	Low / Moderate / Good
Physical Activity	None / Light / Moderate
Mood	Calm / Happy / Irritable / Confused
Energy Level	Low / Medium / High

Daily Observations

Use this space to record any changes or important observations. Examples: confusion, dizziness, swelling, breathing difficulty, behavioural changes, or unusual symptoms.

Bowel Movement & Digestion Tracker

Digestive health is important for many patients, especially those with mobility or medication-related issues.

Bowel Movement	Yes / No
Digestive Discomfort	Yes / No
Notes	____________________

Sleep Quality Tracker

Sleep patterns often reveal important health signals.

Sleep Quality	Excellent / Good / Fair / Poor
Night Disturbances	Yes / No
Daytime Drowsiness	Yes / No

Notes:

Hydration & Nutrition Notes

Food and water intake are critical for recovery and health maintenance.

Meals Consumed Today:
Breakfast / Lunch / Dinner / Snacks

Hydration Level:
Low / Moderate / Good

Notes:

Warning Signs to Watch

Contact a healthcare professional if you notice:

- Sudden confusion or memory changes
- Difficulty breathing
- High fever
- Severe pain
- Persistent dizziness or weakness
- Unusual swelling

If symptoms appear serious, seek medical attention immediately.

Daily Health & Wellness Log

Date: ________________ Day: 14

Health Indicator	Record / Observation
Blood Pressure	________________
Blood Sugar (if applicable)	________________
Temperature	________________
Pulse / Heart Rate	________________
Pain Level (1–10)	________________
Hours of Sleep	________________
Appetite	Poor / Normal / Good
Hydration	Low / Moderate / Good
Physical Activity	None / Light / Moderate
Mood	Calm / Happy / Irritable / Confused
Energy Level	Low / Medium / High

Daily Observations

Use this space to record any changes or important observations. Examples: confusion, dizziness, swelling, breathing difficulty, behavioural changes, or unusual symptoms.

Bowel Movement & Digestion Tracker

Digestive health is important for many patients, especially those with mobility or medication-related issues.

Bowel Movement	Yes / No
Digestive Discomfort	Yes / No
Notes	________________

Sleep Quality Tracker

Sleep patterns often reveal important health signals.

Sleep Quality	Excellent / Good / Fair / Poor
Night Disturbances	Yes / No
Daytime Drowsiness	Yes / No

Notes:

Hydration & Nutrition Notes

Food and water intake are critical for recovery and health maintenance.

Meals Consumed Today:
Breakfast / Lunch / Dinner / Snacks

Hydration Level:
Low / Moderate / Good

Notes:

Warning Signs to Watch

Contact a healthcare professional if you notice:

- Sudden confusion or memory changes
- Difficulty breathing
- High fever
- Severe pain
- Persistent dizziness or weakness
- Unusual swelling

If symptoms appear serious, seek medical attention immediately.

Daily Health & Wellness Log

Date: ________________ Day: 15

Health Indicator	Record / Observation
Blood Pressure	________________
Blood Sugar (if applicable)	________________
Temperature	________________
Pulse / Heart Rate	________________
Pain Level (1–10)	________________
Hours of Sleep	________________
Appetite	Poor / Normal / Good
Hydration	Low / Moderate / Good
Physical Activity	None / Light / Moderate
Mood	Calm / Happy / Irritable / Confused
Energy Level	Low / Medium / High

Daily Observations

Use this space to record any changes or important observations. Examples: confusion, dizziness, swelling, breathing difficulty, behavioural changes, or unusual symptoms.

Bowel Movement & Digestion Tracker

Digestive health is important for many patients, especially those with mobility or medication-related issues.

Bowel Movement	Yes / No
Digestive Discomfort	Yes / No
Notes	________________

Sleep Quality Tracker

Sleep patterns often reveal important health signals.

Sleep Quality	**Excellent / Good / Fair / Poor**
Night Disturbances	Yes / No
Daytime Drowsiness	Yes / No

Notes:

Hydration & Nutrition Notes

Food and water intake are critical for recovery and health maintenance.

Meals Consumed Today:
Breakfast / Lunch / Dinner / Snacks

Hydration Level:
Low / Moderate / Good

Notes:

Warning Signs to Watch

Contact a healthcare professional if you notice:

- Sudden confusion or memory changes
- Difficulty breathing
- High fever
- Severe pain
- Persistent dizziness or weakness
- Unusual swelling

If symptoms appear serious, seek medical attention immediately.

Daily Health & Wellness Log

Date: ________________ Day: 16

Health Indicator	Record / Observation
Blood Pressure	________________
Blood Sugar (if applicable)	________________
Temperature	________________
Pulse / Heart Rate	________________
Pain Level (1–10)	________________
Hours of Sleep	________________
Appetite	Poor / Normal / Good
Hydration	Low / Moderate / Good
Physical Activity	None / Light / Moderate
Mood	Calm / Happy / Irritable / Confused
Energy Level	Low / Medium / High

Daily Observations

Use this space to record any changes or important observations. Examples: confusion, dizziness, swelling, breathing difficulty, behavioural changes, or unusual symptoms.

Bowel Movement & Digestion Tracker

Digestive health is important for many patients, especially those with mobility or medication-related issues.

Bowel Movement	Yes / No
Digestive Discomfort	Yes / No
Notes	________________

Sleep Quality Tracker

Sleep patterns often reveal important health signals.

Sleep Quality	Excellent / Good / Fair / Poor
Night Disturbances	Yes / No
Daytime Drowsiness	Yes / No

Notes:

Hydration & Nutrition Notes

Food and water intake are critical for recovery and health maintenance.

Meals Consumed Today:
Breakfast / Lunch / Dinner / Snacks

Hydration Level:
Low / Moderate / Good

Notes:

Warning Signs to Watch

Contact a healthcare professional if you notice:

- Sudden confusion or memory changes
- Difficulty breathing
- High fever
- Severe pain
- Persistent dizziness or weakness
- Unusual swelling

If symptoms appear serious, seek medical attention immediately.

Daily Health & Wellness Log

Date: ________________ Day: 17

Health Indicator	Record / Observation
Blood Pressure	________________
Blood Sugar (if applicable)	________________
Temperature	________________
Pulse / Heart Rate	________________
Pain Level (1–10)	________________
Hours of Sleep	________________
Appetite	Poor / Normal / Good
Hydration	Low / Moderate / Good
Physical Activity	None / Light / Moderate
Mood	Calm / Happy / Irritable / Confused
Energy Level	Low / Medium / High

Daily Observations

Use this space to record any changes or important observations. Examples: confusion, dizziness, swelling, breathing difficulty, behavioural changes, or unusual symptoms.

Bowel Movement & Digestion Tracker

Digestive health is important for many patients, especially those with mobility or medication-related issues.

Bowel Movement	Yes / No
Digestive Discomfort	Yes / No
Notes	________________

Sleep Quality Tracker

Sleep patterns often reveal important health signals.

Sleep Quality	**Excellent / Good / Fair / Poor**
Night Disturbances	Yes / No
Daytime Drowsiness	Yes / No

Notes:

____

____

Hydration & Nutrition Notes

Food and water intake are critical for recovery and health maintenance.

Meals Consumed Today:
Breakfast / Lunch / Dinner / Snacks

Hydration Level:
Low / Moderate / Good

Notes:

____

____

Warning Signs to Watch

Contact a healthcare professional if you notice:

- Sudden confusion or memory changes
- Difficulty breathing
- High fever
- Severe pain
- Persistent dizziness or weakness
- Unusual swelling

If symptoms appear serious, seek medical attention immediately.

Daily Health & Wellness Log

Date: ________________ Day: 18

Health Indicator	Record / Observation
Blood Pressure	________________
Blood Sugar (if applicable)	________________
Temperature	________________
Pulse / Heart Rate	________________
Pain Level (1–10)	________________
Hours of Sleep	________________
Appetite	Poor / Normal / Good
Hydration	Low / Moderate / Good
Physical Activity	None / Light / Moderate
Mood	Calm / Happy / Irritable / Confused
Energy Level	Low / Medium / High

Daily Observations

Use this space to record any changes or important observations. Examples: confusion, dizziness, swelling, breathing difficulty, behavioural changes, or unusual symptoms.

Bowel Movement & Digestion Tracker

Digestive health is important for many patients, especially those with mobility or medication-related issues.

Bowel Movement	Yes / No
Digestive Discomfort	Yes / No
Notes	________________

Sleep Quality Tracker

Sleep patterns often reveal important health signals.

Sleep Quality	**Excellent / Good / Fair / Poor**
Night Disturbances	Yes / No
Daytime Drowsiness	Yes / No

Notes:

Hydration & Nutrition Notes

Food and water intake are critical for recovery and health maintenance.

Meals Consumed Today:
Breakfast / Lunch / Dinner / Snacks

Hydration Level:
Low / Moderate / Good

Notes:

Warning Signs to Watch

Contact a healthcare professional if you notice:

- Sudden confusion or memory changes
- Difficulty breathing
- High fever
- Severe pain
- Persistent dizziness or weakness
- Unusual swelling

If symptoms appear serious, seek medical attention immediately.

Daily Health & Wellness Log

Date: ________________ Day: 19

Health Indicator	Record / Observation
Blood Pressure	____________________
Blood Sugar (if applicable)	____________________
Temperature	____________________
Pulse / Heart Rate	____________________
Pain Level (1–10)	____________________
Hours of Sleep	____________________
Appetite	Poor / Normal / Good
Hydration	Low / Moderate / Good
Physical Activity	None / Light / Moderate
Mood	Calm / Happy / Irritable / Confused
Energy Level	Low / Medium / High

Daily Observations

Use this space to record any changes or important observations. Examples: confusion, dizziness, swelling, breathing difficulty, behavioural changes, or unusual symptoms.

Bowel Movement & Digestion Tracker

Digestive health is important for many patients, especially those with mobility or medication-related issues.

Bowel Movement	Yes / No
Digestive Discomfort	Yes / No
Notes	____________________

Sleep Quality Tracker

Sleep patterns often reveal important health signals.

Sleep Quality	**Excellent / Good / Fair / Poor**
Night Disturbances	Yes / No
Daytime Drowsiness	Yes / No

Notes:

Hydration & Nutrition Notes

Food and water intake are critical for recovery and health maintenance.

Meals Consumed Today:
Breakfast / Lunch / Dinner / Snacks

Hydration Level:
Low / Moderate / Good

Notes:

Warning Signs to Watch

Contact a healthcare professional if you notice:

- Sudden confusion or memory changes
- Difficulty breathing
- High fever
- Severe pain
- Persistent dizziness or weakness
- Unusual swelling

If symptoms appear serious, seek medical attention immediately.

Daily Health & Wellness Log

Date: ________________ Day: 20

Health Indicator	Record / Observation
Blood Pressure	________________
Blood Sugar (if applicable)	________________
Temperature	________________
Pulse / Heart Rate	________________
Pain Level (1–10)	________________
Hours of Sleep	________________
Appetite	Poor / Normal / Good
Hydration	Low / Moderate / Good
Physical Activity	None / Light / Moderate
Mood	Calm / Happy / Irritable / Confused
Energy Level	Low / Medium / High

Daily Observations

Use this space to record any changes or important observations. Examples: confusion, dizziness, swelling, breathing difficulty, behavioural changes, or unusual symptoms.

Bowel Movement & Digestion Tracker

Digestive health is important for many patients, especially those with mobility or medication-related issues.

Bowel Movement	Yes / No
Digestive Discomfort	Yes / No
Notes	________________

Sleep Quality Tracker

Sleep patterns often reveal important health signals.

Sleep Quality	**Excellent / Good / Fair / Poor**
Night Disturbances	Yes / No
Daytime Drowsiness	Yes / No

Notes:

Hydration & Nutrition Notes

Food and water intake are critical for recovery and health maintenance.

Meals Consumed Today:
Breakfast / Lunch / Dinner / Snacks

Hydration Level:
Low / Moderate / Good

Notes:

Warning Signs to Watch

Contact a healthcare professional if you notice:

- Sudden confusion or memory changes
- Difficulty breathing
- High fever
- Severe pain
- Persistent dizziness or weakness
- Unusual swelling

If symptoms appear serious, seek medical attention immediately.

Daily Health & Wellness Log

Date: ________________ Day: 21

Health Indicator	Record / Observation
Blood Pressure	____________________
Blood Sugar (if applicable)	____________________
Temperature	____________________
Pulse / Heart Rate	____________________
Pain Level (1–10)	____________________
Hours of Sleep	____________________
Appetite	Poor / Normal / Good
Hydration	Low / Moderate / Good
Physical Activity	None / Light / Moderate
Mood	Calm / Happy / Irritable / Confused
Energy Level	Low / Medium / High

Daily Observations

Use this space to record any changes or important observations. Examples: confusion, dizziness, swelling, breathing difficulty, behavioural changes, or unusual symptoms.

Bowel Movement & Digestion Tracker

Digestive health is important for many patients, especially those with mobility or medication-related issues.

Bowel Movement	Yes / No
Digestive Discomfort	Yes / No
Notes	____________________

Sleep Quality Tracker

Sleep patterns often reveal important health signals.

Sleep Quality	**Excellent / Good / Fair / Poor**
Night Disturbances	Yes / No
Daytime Drowsiness	Yes / No

Notes:

Hydration & Nutrition Notes

Food and water intake are critical for recovery and health maintenance.

Meals Consumed Today:
Breakfast / Lunch / Dinner / Snacks

Hydration Level:
Low / Moderate / Good

Notes:

Warning Signs to Watch

Contact a healthcare professional if you notice:

- Sudden confusion or memory changes
- Difficulty breathing
- High fever
- Severe pain
- Persistent dizziness or weakness
- Unusual swelling

If symptoms appear serious, seek medical attention immediately.

Daily Health & Wellness Log

Date: ________________ Day: 22

Health Indicator	Record / Observation
Blood Pressure	__________________
Blood Sugar (if applicable)	__________________
Temperature	__________________
Pulse / Heart Rate	__________________
Pain Level (1–10)	__________________
Hours of Sleep	__________________
Appetite	Poor / Normal / Good
Hydration	Low / Moderate / Good
Physical Activity	None / Light / Moderate
Mood	Calm / Happy / Irritable / Confused
Energy Level	Low / Medium / High

Daily Observations

Use this space to record any changes or important observations. Examples: confusion, dizziness, swelling, breathing difficulty, behavioural changes, or unusual symptoms.

Bowel Movement & Digestion Tracker

Digestive health is important for many patients, especially those with mobility or medication-related issues.

Bowel Movement	Yes / No
Digestive Discomfort	Yes / No
Notes	__________________

Sleep Quality Tracker

Sleep patterns often reveal important health signals.

Sleep Quality	**Excellent / Good / Fair / Poor**
Night Disturbances	Yes / No
Daytime Drowsiness	Yes / No

Notes:

Hydration & Nutrition Notes

Food and water intake are critical for recovery and health maintenance.

Meals Consumed Today:
Breakfast / Lunch / Dinner / Snacks

Hydration Level:
Low / Moderate / Good

Notes:

Warning Signs to Watch

Contact a healthcare professional if you notice:

- Sudden confusion or memory changes
- Difficulty breathing
- High fever
- Severe pain
- Persistent dizziness or weakness
- Unusual swelling

If symptoms appear serious, seek medical attention immediately.

Daily Health & Wellness Log

Date: ________________ Day: 23

Health Indicator	Record / Observation
Blood Pressure	________________
Blood Sugar (if applicable)	________________
Temperature	________________
Pulse / Heart Rate	________________
Pain Level (1–10)	________________
Hours of Sleep	________________
Appetite	Poor / Normal / Good
Hydration	Low / Moderate / Good
Physical Activity	None / Light / Moderate
Mood	Calm / Happy / Irritable / Confused
Energy Level	Low / Medium / High

Daily Observations

Use this space to record any changes or important observations. Examples: confusion, dizziness, swelling, breathing difficulty, behavioural changes, or unusual symptoms.

Bowel Movement & Digestion Tracker

Digestive health is important for many patients, especially those with mobility or medication-related issues.

Bowel Movement	Yes / No
Digestive Discomfort	Yes / No
Notes	________________

Sleep Quality Tracker

Sleep patterns often reveal important health signals.

Sleep Quality	Excellent / Good / Fair / Poor
Night Disturbances	Yes / No
Daytime Drowsiness	Yes / No

Notes:

Hydration & Nutrition Notes

Food and water intake are critical for recovery and health maintenance.

Meals Consumed Today:
Breakfast / Lunch / Dinner / Snacks

Hydration Level:
Low / Moderate / Good

Notes:

Warning Signs to Watch

Contact a healthcare professional if you notice:

- Sudden confusion or memory changes
- Difficulty breathing
- High fever
- Severe pain
- Persistent dizziness or weakness
- Unusual swelling

If symptoms appear serious, seek medical attention immediately.

Daily Health & Wellness Log

Date: _______________ Day: 24

Health Indicator	Record / Observation
Blood Pressure	_________________
Blood Sugar (if applicable)	_________________
Temperature	_________________
Pulse / Heart Rate	_________________
Pain Level (1–10)	_________________
Hours of Sleep	_________________
Appetite	Poor / Normal / Good
Hydration	Low / Moderate / Good
Physical Activity	None / Light / Moderate
Mood	Calm / Happy / Irritable / Confused
Energy Level	Low / Medium / High

Daily Observations

Use this space to record any changes or important observations. Examples: confusion, dizziness, swelling, breathing difficulty, behavioural changes, or unusual symptoms.

Bowel Movement & Digestion Tracker

Digestive health is important for many patients, especially those with mobility or medication-related issues.

Bowel Movement	Yes / No
Digestive Discomfort	Yes / No
Notes	_________________

Sleep Quality Tracker

Sleep patterns often reveal important health signals.

Sleep Quality	Excellent / Good / Fair / Poor
Night Disturbances	Yes / No
Daytime Drowsiness	Yes / No

Notes:

Hydration & Nutrition Notes

Food and water intake are critical for recovery and health maintenance.

Meals Consumed Today:
Breakfast / Lunch / Dinner / Snacks

Hydration Level:
Low / Moderate / Good

Notes:

Warning Signs to Watch

Contact a healthcare professional if you notice:

- Sudden confusion or memory changes
- Difficulty breathing
- High fever
- Severe pain
- Persistent dizziness or weakness
- Unusual swelling

If symptoms appear serious, seek medical attention immediately.

Daily Health & Wellness Log

Date: ________________ Day: 25

Health Indicator	Record / Observation
Blood Pressure	____________________
Blood Sugar (if applicable)	____________________
Temperature	____________________
Pulse / Heart Rate	____________________
Pain Level (1–10)	____________________
Hours of Sleep	____________________
Appetite	Poor / Normal / Good
Hydration	Low / Moderate / Good
Physical Activity	None / Light / Moderate
Mood	Calm / Happy / Irritable / Confused
Energy Level	Low / Medium / High

Daily Observations

Use this space to record any changes or important observations. Examples: confusion, dizziness, swelling, breathing difficulty, behavioural changes, or unusual symptoms.

Bowel Movement & Digestion Tracker

Digestive health is important for many patients, especially those with mobility or medication-related issues.

Bowel Movement	Yes / No
Digestive Discomfort	Yes / No
Notes	____________________

Sleep Quality Tracker

Sleep patterns often reveal important health signals.

Sleep Quality	Excellent / Good / Fair / Poor
Night Disturbances	Yes / No
Daytime Drowsiness	Yes / No

Notes:

Hydration & Nutrition Notes

Food and water intake are critical for recovery and health maintenance.

Meals Consumed Today:
Breakfast / Lunch / Dinner / Snacks

Hydration Level:
Low / Moderate / Good

Notes:

Warning Signs to Watch

Contact a healthcare professional if you notice:

- Sudden confusion or memory changes
- Difficulty breathing
- High fever
- Severe pain
- Persistent dizziness or weakness
- Unusual swelling

If symptoms appear serious, seek medical attention immediately.

Daily Health & Wellness Log

Date: ________________ Day: 26

Health Indicator	Record / Observation
Blood Pressure	________________
Blood Sugar (if applicable)	________________
Temperature	________________
Pulse / Heart Rate	________________
Pain Level (1–10)	________________
Hours of Sleep	________________
Appetite	Poor / Normal / Good
Hydration	Low / Moderate / Good
Physical Activity	None / Light / Moderate
Mood	Calm / Happy / Irritable / Confused
Energy Level	Low / Medium / High

Daily Observations

Use this space to record any changes or important observations. Examples: confusion, dizziness, swelling, breathing difficulty, behavioural changes, or unusual symptoms.

Bowel Movement & Digestion Tracker

Digestive health is important for many patients, especially those with mobility or medication-related issues.

Bowel Movement	Yes / No
Digestive Discomfort	Yes / No
Notes	________________

Sleep Quality Tracker

Sleep patterns often reveal important health signals.

Sleep Quality	**Excellent / Good / Fair / Poor**
Night Disturbances	Yes / No
Daytime Drowsiness	Yes / No

Notes:

Hydration & Nutrition Notes

Food and water intake are critical for recovery and health maintenance.

Meals Consumed Today:
Breakfast / Lunch / Dinner / Snacks

Hydration Level:
Low / Moderate / Good

Notes:

Warning Signs to Watch

Contact a healthcare professional if you notice:

- Sudden confusion or memory changes
- Difficulty breathing
- High fever
- Severe pain
- Persistent dizziness or weakness
- Unusual swelling

If symptoms appear serious, seek medical attention immediately.

Daily Health & Wellness Log

Date: ________________ Day: 27

Health Indicator	Record / Observation
Blood Pressure	________________
Blood Sugar (if applicable)	________________
Temperature	________________
Pulse / Heart Rate	________________
Pain Level (1–10)	________________
Hours of Sleep	________________
Appetite	Poor / Normal / Good
Hydration	Low / Moderate / Good
Physical Activity	None / Light / Moderate
Mood	Calm / Happy / Irritable / Confused
Energy Level	Low / Medium / High

Daily Observations

Use this space to record any changes or important observations. Examples: confusion, dizziness, swelling, breathing difficulty, behavioural changes, or unusual symptoms.

Bowel Movement & Digestion Tracker

Digestive health is important for many patients, especially those with mobility or medication-related issues.

Bowel Movement	Yes / No
Digestive Discomfort	Yes / No
Notes	________________

Sleep Quality Tracker

Sleep patterns often reveal important health signals.

Sleep Quality	Excellent / Good / Fair / Poor
Night Disturbances	Yes / No
Daytime Drowsiness	Yes / No

Notes:

Hydration & Nutrition Notes

Food and water intake are critical for recovery and health maintenance.

Meals Consumed Today:
Breakfast / Lunch / Dinner / Snacks

Hydration Level:
Low / Moderate / Good

Notes:

Warning Signs to Watch

Contact a healthcare professional if you notice:

- Sudden confusion or memory changes
- Difficulty breathing
- High fever
- Severe pain
- Persistent dizziness or weakness
- Unusual swelling

If symptoms appear serious, seek medical attention immediately.

Daily Health & Wellness Log

Date: ________________ Day: 28

Health Indicator	Record / Observation
Blood Pressure	__________________
Blood Sugar (if applicable)	__________________
Temperature	__________________
Pulse / Heart Rate	__________________
Pain Level (1–10)	__________________
Hours of Sleep	__________________
Appetite	Poor / Normal / Good
Hydration	Low / Moderate / Good
Physical Activity	None / Light / Moderate
Mood	Calm / Happy / Irritable / Confused
Energy Level	Low / Medium / High

Daily Observations

Use this space to record any changes or important observations. Examples: confusion, dizziness, swelling, breathing difficulty, behavioural changes, or unusual symptoms.

Bowel Movement & Digestion Tracker

Digestive health is important for many patients, especially those with mobility or medication-related issues.

Bowel Movement	Yes / No
Digestive Discomfort	Yes / No
Notes	__________________

Sleep Quality Tracker

Sleep patterns often reveal important health signals.

Sleep Quality	**Excellent / Good / Fair / Poor**
Night Disturbances	Yes / No
Daytime Drowsiness	Yes / No

Notes:

Hydration & Nutrition Notes

Food and water intake are critical for recovery and health maintenance.

Meals Consumed Today:
Breakfast / Lunch / Dinner / Snacks

Hydration Level:
Low / Moderate / Good

Notes:

Warning Signs to Watch

Contact a healthcare professional if you notice:

- Sudden confusion or memory changes
- Difficulty breathing
- High fever
- Severe pain
- Persistent dizziness or weakness
- Unusual swelling

If symptoms appear serious, seek medical attention immediately.

Daily Health & Wellness Log

Date: ________________ Day: 29

Health Indicator	Record / Observation
Blood Pressure	________________
Blood Sugar (if applicable)	________________
Temperature	________________
Pulse / Heart Rate	________________
Pain Level (1–10)	________________
Hours of Sleep	________________
Appetite	Poor / Normal / Good
Hydration	Low / Moderate / Good
Physical Activity	None / Light / Moderate
Mood	Calm / Happy / Irritable / Confused
Energy Level	Low / Medium / High

Daily Observations

Use this space to record any changes or important observations. Examples: confusion, dizziness, swelling, breathing difficulty, behavioural changes, or unusual symptoms.

Bowel Movement & Digestion Tracker

Digestive health is important for many patients, especially those with mobility or medication-related issues.

Bowel Movement	Yes / No
Digestive Discomfort	Yes / No
Notes	________________

Sleep Quality Tracker

Sleep patterns often reveal important health signals.

Sleep Quality	**Excellent / Good / Fair / Poor**
Night Disturbances	Yes / No
Daytime Drowsiness	Yes / No

Notes:

Hydration & Nutrition Notes

Food and water intake are critical for recovery and health maintenance.

Meals Consumed Today:
Breakfast / Lunch / Dinner / Snacks

Hydration Level:
Low / Moderate / Good

Notes:

Warning Signs to Watch

Contact a healthcare professional if you notice:

- Sudden confusion or memory changes
- Difficulty breathing
- High fever
- Severe pain
- Persistent dizziness or weakness
- Unusual swelling

If symptoms appear serious, seek medical attention immediately.

Section 4
Mood & Behaviour Tracker

Changes in mood and behaviour can often provide early clues about a person's physical or emotional health. For individuals living with memory loss, neurological conditions, or chronic illness, these changes may occur gradually or unexpectedly.

By keeping a simple record of mood, behaviour patterns, and triggers, caregivers may notice trends that can help healthcare professionals better understand the person's condition and adjust treatment if necessary.

This section allows caregivers to document emotional state, behavioural changes, confusion episodes, agitation, and other observations that may be important over time.

Try to record observations at least once per day or whenever noticeable changes occur.

Daily Mood & Behaviour Log

Date: ______________________

Observation Category	Record / Notes
Overall Mood	Happy / Calm / Neutral / Irritable / Sad
Anxiety Level	None / Mild / Moderate / High
Confusion or Memory Issues	None / Mild / Moderate / Severe
Agitation or Restlessness	None / Mild / Moderate / Severe
Social Interaction	Engaged / Quiet / Withdrawn
Communication Ability	Normal / Slower / Difficulty Speaking
Cooperation With Care	Cooperative / Resistant
Sleep Disturbance	Yes / No

Behaviour Changes Observed

Describe any unusual or new behaviours noticed today.

Examples: wandering, repeated questions, sudden anger, unusual quietness, confusion about time or place.

Possible Triggers

If a behavioural change occurred, note anything that may have triggered it.

Examples: loud environment, fatigue, medication change, unfamiliar surroundings.

Activities Today

Sometimes activities can affect mood or behaviour.

Activities completed today:

☐ Light exercise
☐ Conversation with family or friends
☐ Reading or puzzles
☐ Music or relaxation
☐ Outdoor time
☐ Doctor visit
☐ Other: __________________

Notes:

____

____

Calming Strategies Used

If the person became upset, what helped calm them?

Examples: reassurance, quiet environment, music, rest.

____

____

____

Caregiver Notes

Record anything important you may want to discuss with a doctor or healthcare provider.

____

____

____

____

Daily Mood & Behaviour Log

Date: ______________________

Observation Category	Record / Notes
Overall Mood	Happy / Calm / Neutral / Irritable / Sad
Anxiety Level	None / Mild / Moderate / High
Confusion or Memory Issues	None / Mild / Moderate / Severe
Agitation or Restlessness	None / Mild / Moderate / Severe
Social Interaction	Engaged / Quiet / Withdrawn
Communication Ability	Normal / Slower / Difficulty Speaking
Cooperation With Care	Cooperative / Resistant
Sleep Disturbance	Yes / No

Behaviour Changes Observed

Describe any unusual or new behaviours noticed today.

Examples: wandering, repeated questions, sudden anger, unusual quietness, confusion about time or place.

Possible Triggers

If a behavioural change occurred, note anything that may have triggered it.

Examples: loud environment, fatigue, medication change, unfamiliar surroundings.

Activities Today

Sometimes activities can affect mood or behaviour

.

Activities completed today:

☐ Light exercise
☐ Conversation with family or friends
☐ Reading or puzzles
☐ Music or relaxation
☐ Outdoor time
☐ Doctor visit
☐ Other: ___________________

Notes:

Calming Strategies Used

If the person became upset, what helped calm them?

Examples: reassurance, quiet environment, music, rest.

Caregiver Notes

Record anything important you may want to discuss with a doctor or healthcare provider.

Daily Mood & Behaviour Log

Date: ______________________

Observation Category	Record / Notes
Overall Mood	Happy / Calm / Neutral / Irritable / Sad
Anxiety Level	None / Mild / Moderate / High
Confusion or Memory Issues	None / Mild / Moderate / Severe
Agitation or Restlessness	None / Mild / Moderate / Severe
Social Interaction	Engaged / Quiet / Withdrawn
Communication Ability	Normal / Slower / Difficulty Speaking
Cooperation With Care	Cooperative / Resistant
Sleep Disturbance	Yes / No

Behaviour Changes Observed

Describe any unusual or new behaviours noticed today.

Examples: wandering, repeated questions, sudden anger, unusual quietness, confusion about time or place.

Possible Triggers

If a behavioural change occurred, note anything that may have triggered it.

Examples: loud environment, fatigue, medication change, unfamiliar surroundings.

Activities Today

Sometimes activities can affect mood or behaviour

Activities completed today:

☐ Light exercise
☐ Conversation with family or friends
☐ Reading or puzzles
☐ Music or relaxation
☐ Outdoor time
☐ Doctor visit
☐ Other: ___________________

Notes:

____

____

Calming Strategies Used

If the person became upset, what helped calm them?

Examples: reassurance, quiet environment, music, rest.

____

____

____

Caregiver Notes

Record anything important you may want to discuss with a doctor or healthcare provider.

____

____

____

____

Daily Mood & Behaviour Log

Date: ______________________

Observation Category	Record / Notes
Overall Mood	Happy / Calm / Neutral / Irritable / Sad
Anxiety Level	None / Mild / Moderate / High
Confusion or Memory Issues	None / Mild / Moderate / Severe
Agitation or Restlessness	None / Mild / Moderate / Severe
Social Interaction	Engaged / Quiet / Withdrawn
Communication Ability	Normal / Slower / Difficulty Speaking
Cooperation With Care	Cooperative / Resistant
Sleep Disturbance	Yes / No

Behaviour Changes Observed

Describe any unusual or new behaviours noticed today.

Examples: wandering, repeated questions, sudden anger, unusual quietness, confusion about time or place.

Possible Triggers

If a behavioural change occurred, note anything that may have triggered it.

Examples: loud environment, fatigue, medication change, unfamiliar surroundings.

Activities Today

Sometimes activities can affect mood or behaviour

Activities completed today:

☐ Light exercise
☐ Conversation with family or friends
☐ Reading or puzzles
☐ Music or relaxation
☐ Outdoor time
☐ Doctor visit
☐ Other: ___________________

Notes:

____

____

Calming Strategies Used

If the person became upset, what helped calm them?

Examples: reassurance, quiet environment, music, rest.

____

____

____

Caregiver Notes

Record anything important you may want to discuss with a doctor or healthcare provider.

____

____

____

____

Daily Mood & Behaviour Log

Date: ______________________

Observation Category	Record / Notes
Overall Mood	Happy / Calm / Neutral / Irritable / Sad
Anxiety Level	None / Mild / Moderate / High
Confusion or Memory Issues	None / Mild / Moderate / Severe
Agitation or Restlessness	None / Mild / Moderate / Severe
Social Interaction	Engaged / Quiet / Withdrawn
Communication Ability	Normal / Slower / Difficulty Speaking
Cooperation With Care	Cooperative / Resistant
Sleep Disturbance	Yes / No

Behaviour Changes Observed

Describe any unusual or new behaviours noticed today.

Examples: wandering, repeated questions, sudden anger, unusual quietness, confusion about time or place.

Possible Triggers

If a behavioural change occurred, note anything that may have triggered it.

Examples: loud environment, fatigue, medication change, unfamiliar surroundings.

Activities Today

Sometimes activities can affect mood or behaviour

Activities completed today:

☐ Light exercise
☐ Conversation with family or friends
☐ Reading or puzzles
☐ Music or relaxation
☐ Outdoor time
☐ Doctor visit
☐ Other: ________________

Notes:

Calming Strategies Used

If the person became upset, what helped calm them?

Examples: reassurance, quiet environment, music, rest.

Caregiver Notes

Record anything important you may want to discuss with a doctor or healthcare provider.

Daily Mood & Behaviour Log

Date: ______________________

Observation Category	Record / Notes
Overall Mood	Happy / Calm / Neutral / Irritable / Sad
Anxiety Level	None / Mild / Moderate / High
Confusion or Memory Issues	None / Mild / Moderate / Severe
Agitation or Restlessness	None / Mild / Moderate / Severe
Social Interaction	Engaged / Quiet / Withdrawn
Communication Ability	Normal / Slower / Difficulty Speaking
Cooperation With Care	Cooperative / Resistant
Sleep Disturbance	Yes / No

Behaviour Changes Observed

Describe any unusual or new behaviours noticed today.

Examples: wandering, repeated questions, sudden anger, unusual quietness, confusion about time or place.

Possible Triggers

If a behavioural change occurred, note anything that may have triggered it.

Examples: loud environment, fatigue, medication change, unfamiliar surroundings.

Activities Today

Sometimes activities can affect mood or behaviour

Activities completed today:

☐ Light exercise
☐ Conversation with family or friends
☐ Reading or puzzles
☐ Music or relaxation
☐ Outdoor time
☐ Doctor visit
☐ Other: __________________

Notes:

Calming Strategies Used

If the person became upset, what helped calm them?

Examples: reassurance, quiet environment, music, rest.

Caregiver Notes

Record anything important you may want to discuss with a doctor or healthcare provider.

Daily Mood & Behaviour Log

Date: ______________________

Observation Category	Record / Notes
Overall Mood	Happy / Calm / Neutral / Irritable / Sad
Anxiety Level	None / Mild / Moderate / High
Confusion or Memory Issues	None / Mild / Moderate / Severe
Agitation or Restlessness	None / Mild / Moderate / Severe
Social Interaction	Engaged / Quiet / Withdrawn
Communication Ability	Normal / Slower / Difficulty Speaking
Cooperation With Care	Cooperative / Resistant
Sleep Disturbance	Yes / No

Behaviour Changes Observed

Describe any unusual or new behaviours noticed today.

Examples: wandering, repeated questions, sudden anger, unusual quietness, confusion about time or place.

Possible Triggers

If a behavioural change occurred, note anything that may have triggered it.

Examples: loud environment, fatigue, medication change, unfamiliar surroundings.

Activities Today

Sometimes activities can affect mood or behaviour

Activities completed today:

☐ Light exercise
☐ Conversation with family or friends
☐ Reading or puzzles
☐ Music or relaxation
☐ Outdoor time
☐ Doctor visit
☐ Other: ________________

Notes:

____

____

Calming Strategies Used

If the person became upset, what helped calm them?

Examples: reassurance, quiet environment, music, rest.

____

____

____

Caregiver Notes

Record anything important you may want to discuss with a doctor or healthcare provider.

____

____

____

____

Daily Mood & Behaviour Log

Date: ______________________

Observation Category	Record / Notes
Overall Mood	Happy / Calm / Neutral / Irritable / Sad
Anxiety Level	None / Mild / Moderate / High
Confusion or Memory Issues	None / Mild / Moderate / Severe
Agitation or Restlessness	None / Mild / Moderate / Severe
Social Interaction	Engaged / Quiet / Withdrawn
Communication Ability	Normal / Slower / Difficulty Speaking
Cooperation With Care	Cooperative / Resistant
Sleep Disturbance	Yes / No

Behaviour Changes Observed

Describe any unusual or new behaviours noticed today.

Examples: wandering, repeated questions, sudden anger, unusual quietness, confusion about time or place.

Possible Triggers

If a behavioural change occurred, note anything that may have triggered it.

Examples: loud environment, fatigue, medication change, unfamiliar surroundings.

Activities Today

Sometimes activities can affect mood or behaviour

Activities completed today:

☐ Light exercise
☐ Conversation with family or friends
☐ Reading or puzzles
☐ Music or relaxation
☐ Outdoor time
☐ Doctor visit
☐ Other: ___________________

Notes:

Calming Strategies Used

If the person became upset, what helped calm them?

Examples: reassurance, quiet environment, music, rest.

Caregiver Notes

Record anything important you may want to discuss with a doctor or healthcare provider.

Daily Mood & Behaviour Log

Date: ______________________

Observation Category	Record / Notes
Overall Mood	Happy / Calm / Neutral / Irritable / Sad
Anxiety Level	None / Mild / Moderate / High
Confusion or Memory Issues	None / Mild / Moderate / Severe
Agitation or Restlessness	None / Mild / Moderate / Severe
Social Interaction	Engaged / Quiet / Withdrawn
Communication Ability	Normal / Slower / Difficulty Speaking
Cooperation With Care	Cooperative / Resistant
Sleep Disturbance	Yes / No

Behaviour Changes Observed

Describe any unusual or new behaviours noticed today.

Examples: wandering, repeated questions, sudden anger, unusual quietness, confusion about time or place.

Possible Triggers

If a behavioural change occurred, note anything that may have triggered it.

Examples: loud environment, fatigue, medication change, unfamiliar surroundings.

Activities Today

Sometimes activities can affect mood or behaviour

Activities completed today:

☐ Light exercise
☐ Conversation with family or friends
☐ Reading or puzzles
☐ Music or relaxation
☐ Outdoor time
☐ Doctor visit
☐ Other: ____________________

Notes:

____

____

Calming Strategies Used

If the person became upset, what helped calm them?

Examples: reassurance, quiet environment, music, rest.

____

____

____

Caregiver Notes

Record anything important you may want to discuss with a doctor or healthcare provider.

____

____

____

____

Daily Mood & Behaviour Log

Date: ______________________

Observation Category	Record / Notes
Overall Mood	Happy / Calm / Neutral / Irritable / Sad
Anxiety Level	None / Mild / Moderate / High
Confusion or Memory Issues	None / Mild / Moderate / Severe
Agitation or Restlessness	None / Mild / Moderate / Severe
Social Interaction	Engaged / Quiet / Withdrawn
Communication Ability	Normal / Slower / Difficulty Speaking
Cooperation With Care	Cooperative / Resistant
Sleep Disturbance	Yes / No

Behaviour Changes Observed

Describe any unusual or new behaviours noticed today.

Examples: wandering, repeated questions, sudden anger, unusual quietness, confusion about time or place.

Possible Triggers

If a behavioural change occurred, note anything that may have triggered it.

Examples: loud environment, fatigue, medication change, unfamiliar surroundings.

Activities Today

Sometimes activities can affect mood or behaviour

Activities completed today:

☐ Light exercise
☐ Conversation with family or friends
☐ Reading or puzzles
☐ Music or relaxation
☐ Outdoor time
☐ Doctor visit
☐ Other: ___________________

Notes:

____

____

Calming Strategies Used

If the person became upset, what helped calm them?

Examples: reassurance, quiet environment, music, rest.

____

____

____

Caregiver Notes

Record anything important you may want to discuss with a doctor or healthcare provider.

____

____

____

____

Daily Mood & Behaviour Log

Date: ______________________

Observation Category	Record / Notes
Overall Mood	Happy / Calm / Neutral / Irritable / Sad
Anxiety Level	None / Mild / Moderate / High
Confusion or Memory Issues	None / Mild / Moderate / Severe
Agitation or Restlessness	None / Mild / Moderate / Severe
Social Interaction	Engaged / Quiet / Withdrawn
Communication Ability	Normal / Slower / Difficulty Speaking
Cooperation With Care	Cooperative / Resistant
Sleep Disturbance	Yes / No

Behaviour Changes Observed

Describe any unusual or new behaviours noticed today.

Examples: wandering, repeated questions, sudden anger, unusual quietness, confusion about time or place.

Possible Triggers

If a behavioural change occurred, note anything that may have triggered it.

Examples: loud environment, fatigue, medication change, unfamiliar surroundings.

Activities Today

Sometimes activities can affect mood or behaviour

Activities completed today:

☐ Light exercise
☐ Conversation with family or friends
☐ Reading or puzzles
☐ Music or relaxation
☐ Outdoor time
☐ Doctor visit
☐ Other: ________________

Notes:

Calming Strategies Used

If the person became upset, what helped calm them?

Examples: reassurance, quiet environment, music, rest.

Caregiver Notes

Record anything important you may want to discuss with a doctor or healthcare provider.

Daily Mood & Behaviour Log

Date: ______________________

Observation Category	Record / Notes
Overall Mood	Happy / Calm / Neutral / Irritable / Sad
Anxiety Level	None / Mild / Moderate / High
Confusion or Memory Issues	None / Mild / Moderate / Severe
Agitation or Restlessness	None / Mild / Moderate / Severe
Social Interaction	Engaged / Quiet / Withdrawn
Communication Ability	Normal / Slower / Difficulty Speaking
Cooperation With Care	Cooperative / Resistant
Sleep Disturbance	Yes / No

Behaviour Changes Observed

Describe any unusual or new behaviours noticed today.

Examples: wandering, repeated questions, sudden anger, unusual quietness, confusion about time or place.

Possible Triggers

If a behavioural change occurred, note anything that may have triggered it.

Examples: loud environment, fatigue, medication change, unfamiliar surroundings.

Activities Today

Sometimes activities can affect mood or behaviour

Activities completed today:

☐ Light exercise
☐ Conversation with family or friends
☐ Reading or puzzles
☐ Music or relaxation
☐ Outdoor time
☐ Doctor visit
☐ Other: __________________

Notes:

Calming Strategies Used

If the person became upset, what helped calm them?

Examples: reassurance, quiet environment, music, rest.

Caregiver Notes

Record anything important you may want to discuss with a doctor or healthcare provider.

Daily Mood & Behaviour Log

Date: ______________________

Observation Category	Record / Notes
Overall Mood	Happy / Calm / Neutral / Irritable / Sad
Anxiety Level	None / Mild / Moderate / High
Confusion or Memory Issues	None / Mild / Moderate / Severe
Agitation or Restlessness	None / Mild / Moderate / Severe
Social Interaction	Engaged / Quiet / Withdrawn
Communication Ability	Normal / Slower / Difficulty Speaking
Cooperation With Care	Cooperative / Resistant
Sleep Disturbance	Yes / No

Behaviour Changes Observed

Describe any unusual or new behaviours noticed today.

Examples: wandering, repeated questions, sudden anger, unusual quietness, confusion about time or place.

Possible Triggers

If a behavioural change occurred, note anything that may have triggered it.

Examples: loud environment, fatigue, medication change, unfamiliar surroundings.

Activities Today

Sometimes activities can affect mood or behaviour

Activities completed today:

☐ Light exercise
☐ Conversation with family or friends
☐ Reading or puzzles
☐ Music or relaxation
☐ Outdoor time
☐ Doctor visit
☐ Other: ___________________

Notes:

Calming Strategies Used

If the person became upset, what helped calm them?

Examples: reassurance, quiet environment, music, rest.

Caregiver Notes

Record anything important you may want to discuss with a doctor or healthcare provider.

Daily Mood & Behaviour Log

Date: ______________________

Observation Category	Record / Notes
Overall Mood	Happy / Calm / Neutral / Irritable / Sad
Anxiety Level	None / Mild / Moderate / High
Confusion or Memory Issues	None / Mild / Moderate / Severe
Agitation or Restlessness	None / Mild / Moderate / Severe
Social Interaction	Engaged / Quiet / Withdrawn
Communication Ability	Normal / Slower / Difficulty Speaking
Cooperation With Care	Cooperative / Resistant
Sleep Disturbance	Yes / No

Behaviour Changes Observed

Describe any unusual or new behaviours noticed today.

Examples: wandering, repeated questions, sudden anger, unusual quietness, confusion about time or place.

Possible Triggers

If a behavioural change occurred, note anything that may have triggered it.

Examples: loud environment, fatigue, medication change, unfamiliar surroundings.

Activities Today

Sometimes activities can affect mood or behaviour

Activities completed today:

☐ Light exercise
☐ Conversation with family or friends
☐ Reading or puzzles
☐ Music or relaxation
☐ Outdoor time
☐ Doctor visit
☐ Other: ___________________

Notes:

Calming Strategies Used

If the person became upset, what helped calm them?

Examples: reassurance, quiet environment, music, rest.

Caregiver Notes

Record anything important you may want to discuss with a doctor or healthcare provider.

Daily Mood & Behaviour Log

Date: ______________________

Observation Category	Record / Notes
Overall Mood	Happy / Calm / Neutral / Irritable / Sad
Anxiety Level	None / Mild / Moderate / High
Confusion or Memory Issues	None / Mild / Moderate / Severe
Agitation or Restlessness	None / Mild / Moderate / Severe
Social Interaction	Engaged / Quiet / Withdrawn
Communication Ability	Normal / Slower / Difficulty Speaking
Cooperation With Care	Cooperative / Resistant
Sleep Disturbance	Yes / No

Behaviour Changes Observed

Describe any unusual or new behaviours noticed today.

Examples: wandering, repeated questions, sudden anger, unusual quietness, confusion about time or place.

Possible Triggers

If a behavioural change occurred, note anything that may have triggered it.

Examples: loud environment, fatigue, medication change, unfamiliar surroundings.

Activities Today

Sometimes activities can affect mood or behaviour

Activities completed today:

☐ Light exercise
☐ Conversation with family or friends
☐ Reading or puzzles
☐ Music or relaxation
☐ Outdoor time
☐ Doctor visit
☐ Other: ___________________

Notes:

Calming Strategies Used

If the person became upset, what helped calm them?

Examples: reassurance, quiet environment, music, rest.

Caregiver Notes

Record anything important you may want to discuss with a doctor or healthcare provider.

Daily Mood & Behaviour Log

Date: ______________________

Observation Category	Record / Notes
Overall Mood	Happy / Calm / Neutral / Irritable / Sad
Anxiety Level	None / Mild / Moderate / High
Confusion or Memory Issues	None / Mild / Moderate / Severe
Agitation or Restlessness	None / Mild / Moderate / Severe
Social Interaction	Engaged / Quiet / Withdrawn
Communication Ability	Normal / Slower / Difficulty Speaking
Cooperation With Care	Cooperative / Resistant
Sleep Disturbance	Yes / No

Behaviour Changes Observed

Describe any unusual or new behaviours noticed today.

Examples: wandering, repeated questions, sudden anger, unusual quietness, confusion about time or place.

Possible Triggers

If a behavioural change occurred, note anything that may have triggered it.

Examples: loud environment, fatigue, medication change, unfamiliar surroundings.

Activities Today

Sometimes activities can affect mood or behaviour

Activities completed today:

☐ Light exercise
☐ Conversation with family or friends
☐ Reading or puzzles
☐ Music or relaxation
☐ Outdoor time
☐ Doctor visit
☐ Other: ___________________

Notes:

____

____

Calming Strategies Used

If the person became upset, what helped calm them?

Examples: reassurance, quiet environment, music, rest.

____

____

____

Caregiver Notes

Record anything important you may want to discuss with a doctor or healthcare provider.

____

____

____

____

Daily Mood & Behaviour Log

Date: ______________________

Observation Category	Record / Notes
Overall Mood	Happy / Calm / Neutral / Irritable / Sad
Anxiety Level	None / Mild / Moderate / High
Confusion or Memory Issues	None / Mild / Moderate / Severe
Agitation or Restlessness	None / Mild / Moderate / Severe
Social Interaction	Engaged / Quiet / Withdrawn
Communication Ability	Normal / Slower / Difficulty Speaking
Cooperation With Care	Cooperative / Resistant
Sleep Disturbance	Yes / No

Behaviour Changes Observed

Describe any unusual or new behaviours noticed today.

Examples: wandering, repeated questions, sudden anger, unusual quietness, confusion about time or place.

____

____

____

____

Possible Triggers

If a behavioural change occurred, note anything that may have triggered it.

Examples: loud environment, fatigue, medication change, unfamiliar surroundings.

____

____

____

Activities Today

Sometimes activities can affect mood or behaviour

Activities completed today:

☐ Light exercise
☐ Conversation with family or friends
☐ Reading or puzzles
☐ Music or relaxation
☐ Outdoor time
☐ Doctor visit
☐ Other: ____________________

Notes:

____

____

Calming Strategies Used

If the person became upset, what helped calm them?

Examples: reassurance, quiet environment, music, rest.

____

____

____

Caregiver Notes

Record anything important you may want to discuss with a doctor or healthcare provider.

____

____

____

____

Daily Mood & Behaviour Log

Date: ______________________

Observation Category	Record / Notes
Overall Mood	Happy / Calm / Neutral / Irritable / Sad
Anxiety Level	None / Mild / Moderate / High
Confusion or Memory Issues	None / Mild / Moderate / Severe
Agitation or Restlessness	None / Mild / Moderate / Severe
Social Interaction	Engaged / Quiet / Withdrawn
Communication Ability	Normal / Slower / Difficulty Speaking
Cooperation With Care	Cooperative / Resistant
Sleep Disturbance	Yes / No

Behaviour Changes Observed

Describe any unusual or new behaviours noticed today.

Examples: wandering, repeated questions, sudden anger, unusual quietness, confusion about time or place.

Possible Triggers

If a behavioural change occurred, note anything that may have triggered it.

Examples: loud environment, fatigue, medication change, unfamiliar surroundings.

Activities Today

Sometimes activities can affect mood or behaviour

Activities completed today:

☐ Light exercise
☐ Conversation with family or friends
☐ Reading or puzzles
☐ Music or relaxation
☐ Outdoor time
☐ Doctor visit
☐ Other: ___________________

Notes:

____

____

Calming Strategies Used

If the person became upset, what helped calm them?

Examples: reassurance, quiet environment, music, rest.

____

____

____

Caregiver Notes

Record anything important you may want to discuss with a doctor or healthcare provider.

____

____

____

____

Daily Mood & Behaviour Log

Date: ______________________

Observation Category	Record / Notes
Overall Mood	Happy / Calm / Neutral / Irritable / Sad
Anxiety Level	None / Mild / Moderate / High
Confusion or Memory Issues	None / Mild / Moderate / Severe
Agitation or Restlessness	None / Mild / Moderate / Severe
Social Interaction	Engaged / Quiet / Withdrawn
Communication Ability	Normal / Slower / Difficulty Speaking
Cooperation With Care	Cooperative / Resistant
Sleep Disturbance	Yes / No

Behaviour Changes Observed

Describe any unusual or new behaviours noticed today.

Examples: wandering, repeated questions, sudden anger, unusual quietness, confusion about time or place.

Possible Triggers

If a behavioural change occurred, note anything that may have triggered it.

Examples: loud environment, fatigue, medication change, unfamiliar surroundings.

Activities Today

Sometimes activities can affect mood or behaviour

Activities completed today:

☐ Light exercise
☐ Conversation with family or friends
☐ Reading or puzzles
☐ Music or relaxation
☐ Outdoor time
☐ Doctor visit
☐ Other: ___________________

Notes:

____

____

Calming Strategies Used

If the person became upset, what helped calm them?

Examples: reassurance, quiet environment, music, rest.

____

____

____

Caregiver Notes

Record anything important you may want to discuss with a doctor or healthcare provider.

____

____

____

____

Daily Mood & Behaviour Log

Date: ____________________

Observation Category	Record / Notes
Overall Mood	Happy / Calm / Neutral / Irritable / Sad
Anxiety Level	None / Mild / Moderate / High
Confusion or Memory Issues	None / Mild / Moderate / Severe
Agitation or Restlessness	None / Mild / Moderate / Severe
Social Interaction	Engaged / Quiet / Withdrawn
Communication Ability	Normal / Slower / Difficulty Speaking
Cooperation With Care	Cooperative / Resistant
Sleep Disturbance	Yes / No

Behaviour Changes Observed

Describe any unusual or new behaviours noticed today.

Examples: wandering, repeated questions, sudden anger, unusual quietness, confusion about time or place.

Possible Triggers

If a behavioural change occurred, note anything that may have triggered it.

Examples: loud environment, fatigue, medication change, unfamiliar surroundings.

Activities Today

Sometimes activities can affect mood or behaviour

Activities completed today:

☐ Light exercise
☐ Conversation with family or friends
☐ Reading or puzzles
☐ Music or relaxation
☐ Outdoor time
☐ Doctor visit
☐ Other: ___________________

Notes:

____

____

Calming Strategies Used

If the person became upset, what helped calm them?

Examples: reassurance, quiet environment, music, rest.

____

____

____

Caregiver Notes

Record anything important you may want to discuss with a doctor or healthcare provider.

____

____

____

____

Daily Mood & Behaviour Log

Date: ______________________

Observation Category	Record / Notes
Overall Mood	Happy / Calm / Neutral / Irritable / Sad
Anxiety Level	None / Mild / Moderate / High
Confusion or Memory Issues	None / Mild / Moderate / Severe
Agitation or Restlessness	None / Mild / Moderate / Severe
Social Interaction	Engaged / Quiet / Withdrawn
Communication Ability	Normal / Slower / Difficulty Speaking
Cooperation With Care	Cooperative / Resistant
Sleep Disturbance	Yes / No

Behaviour Changes Observed

Describe any unusual or new behaviours noticed today.

Examples: wandering, repeated questions, sudden anger, unusual quietness, confusion about time or place.

Possible Triggers

If a behavioural change occurred, note anything that may have triggered it.

Examples: loud environment, fatigue, medication change, unfamiliar surroundings.

Activities Today

Sometimes activities can affect mood or behaviour

Activities completed today:

☐ Light exercise
☐ Conversation with family or friends
☐ Reading or puzzles
☐ Music or relaxation
☐ Outdoor time
☐ Doctor visit
☐ Other: ________________

Notes:

____

____

Calming Strategies Used

If the person became upset, what helped calm them?

Examples: reassurance, quiet environment, music, rest.

____

____

____

Caregiver Notes

Record anything important you may want to discuss with a doctor or healthcare provider.

____

____

____

____

Daily Mood & Behaviour Log

Date: ______________________

Observation Category	Record / Notes
Overall Mood	Happy / Calm / Neutral / Irritable / Sad
Anxiety Level	None / Mild / Moderate / High
Confusion or Memory Issues	None / Mild / Moderate / Severe
Agitation or Restlessness	None / Mild / Moderate / Severe
Social Interaction	Engaged / Quiet / Withdrawn
Communication Ability	Normal / Slower / Difficulty Speaking
Cooperation With Care	Cooperative / Resistant
Sleep Disturbance	Yes / No

Behaviour Changes Observed

Describe any unusual or new behaviours noticed today.

Examples: wandering, repeated questions, sudden anger, unusual quietness, confusion about time or place.

Possible Triggers

If a behavioural change occurred, note anything that may have triggered it.

Examples: loud environment, fatigue, medication change, unfamiliar surroundings.

Activities Today

Sometimes activities can affect mood or behaviour

Activities completed today:

☐ Light exercise
☐ Conversation with family or friends
☐ Reading or puzzles
☐ Music or relaxation
☐ Outdoor time
☐ Doctor visit
☐ Other: ___________________

Notes:

____

____

Calming Strategies Used

If the person became upset, what helped calm them?

Examples: reassurance, quiet environment, music, rest.

____

____

____

Caregiver Notes

Record anything important you may want to discuss with a doctor or healthcare provider.

____

____

____

____

Daily Mood & Behaviour Log

Date: ______________________

Observation Category	Record / Notes
Overall Mood	Happy / Calm / Neutral / Irritable / Sad
Anxiety Level	None / Mild / Moderate / High
Confusion or Memory Issues	None / Mild / Moderate / Severe
Agitation or Restlessness	None / Mild / Moderate / Severe
Social Interaction	Engaged / Quiet / Withdrawn
Communication Ability	Normal / Slower / Difficulty Speaking
Cooperation With Care	Cooperative / Resistant
Sleep Disturbance	Yes / No

Behaviour Changes Observed

Describe any unusual or new behaviours noticed today.

Examples: wandering, repeated questions, sudden anger, unusual quietness, confusion about time or place.

Possible Triggers

If a behavioural change occurred, note anything that may have triggered it.

Examples: loud environment, fatigue, medication change, unfamiliar surroundings.

Activities Today

Sometimes activities can affect mood or behaviour

Activities completed today:

☐ Light exercise
☐ Conversation with family or friends
☐ Reading or puzzles
☐ Music or relaxation
☐ Outdoor time
☐ Doctor visit
☐ Other: __________________

Notes:

____

____

Calming Strategies Used

If the person became upset, what helped calm them?

Examples: reassurance, quiet environment, music, rest.

____

____

____

Caregiver Notes

Record anything important you may want to discuss with a doctor or healthcare provider.

____

____

____

____

Daily Mood & Behaviour Log

Date: ______________________

Observation Category	Record / Notes
Overall Mood	Happy / Calm / Neutral / Irritable / Sad
Anxiety Level	None / Mild / Moderate / High
Confusion or Memory Issues	None / Mild / Moderate / Severe
Agitation or Restlessness	None / Mild / Moderate / Severe
Social Interaction	Engaged / Quiet / Withdrawn
Communication Ability	Normal / Slower / Difficulty Speaking
Cooperation With Care	Cooperative / Resistant
Sleep Disturbance	Yes / No

Behaviour Changes Observed

Describe any unusual or new behaviours noticed today.

Examples: wandering, repeated questions, sudden anger, unusual quietness, confusion about time or place.

Possible Triggers

If a behavioural change occurred, note anything that may have triggered it.

Examples: loud environment, fatigue, medication change, unfamiliar surroundings.

Activities Today

Sometimes activities can affect mood or behaviour

Activities completed today:

☐ Light exercise
☐ Conversation with family or friends
☐ Reading or puzzles
☐ Music or relaxation
☐ Outdoor time
☐ Doctor visit
☐ Other: ____________________

Notes:

____

____

Calming Strategies Used

If the person became upset, what helped calm them?

Examples: reassurance, quiet environment, music, rest.

____

____

____

Caregiver Notes

Record anything important you may want to discuss with a doctor or healthcare provider.

____

____

____

____

Daily Mood & Behaviour Log

Date: ______________________

Observation Category	Record / Notes
Overall Mood	Happy / Calm / Neutral / Irritable / Sad
Anxiety Level	None / Mild / Moderate / High
Confusion or Memory Issues	None / Mild / Moderate / Severe
Agitation or Restlessness	None / Mild / Moderate / Severe
Social Interaction	Engaged / Quiet / Withdrawn
Communication Ability	Normal / Slower / Difficulty Speaking
Cooperation With Care	Cooperative / Resistant
Sleep Disturbance	Yes / No

Behaviour Changes Observed

Describe any unusual or new behaviours noticed today.

Examples: wandering, repeated questions, sudden anger, unusual quietness, confusion about time or place.

Possible Triggers

If a behavioural change occurred, note anything that may have triggered it.

Examples: loud environment, fatigue, medication change, unfamiliar surroundings.

Activities Today

Sometimes activities can affect mood or behaviour

Activities completed today:

☐ Light exercise
☐ Conversation with family or friends
☐ Reading or puzzles
☐ Music or relaxation
☐ Outdoor time
☐ Doctor visit
☐ Other: ___________________

Notes:

____

____

Calming Strategies Used

If the person became upset, what helped calm them?

Examples: reassurance, quiet environment, music, rest.

____

____

____

Caregiver Notes

Record anything important you may want to discuss with a doctor or healthcare provider.

____

____

____

____

Daily Mood & Behaviour Log

Date: ______________________

Observation Category	Record / Notes
Overall Mood	Happy / Calm / Neutral / Irritable / Sad
Anxiety Level	None / Mild / Moderate / High
Confusion or Memory Issues	None / Mild / Moderate / Severe
Agitation or Restlessness	None / Mild / Moderate / Severe
Social Interaction	Engaged / Quiet / Withdrawn
Communication Ability	Normal / Slower / Difficulty Speaking
Cooperation With Care	Cooperative / Resistant
Sleep Disturbance	Yes / No

Behaviour Changes Observed

Describe any unusual or new behaviours noticed today.

Examples: wandering, repeated questions, sudden anger, unusual quietness, confusion about time or place.

Possible Triggers

If a behavioural change occurred, note anything that may have triggered it.

Examples: loud environment, fatigue, medication change, unfamiliar surroundings.

Activities Today

Sometimes activities can affect mood or behaviour

Activities completed today:

☐ Light exercise
☐ Conversation with family or friends
☐ Reading or puzzles
☐ Music or relaxation
☐ Outdoor time
☐ Doctor visit
☐ Other: ____________________

Notes:

____

____

Calming Strategies Used

If the person became upset, what helped calm them?

Examples: reassurance, quiet environment, music, rest.

____

____

____

Caregiver Notes

Record anything important you may want to discuss with a doctor or healthcare provider.

____

____

____

____

Daily Mood & Behaviour Log

Date: ______________________

Observation Category	Record / Notes
Overall Mood	Happy / Calm / Neutral / Irritable / Sad
Anxiety Level	None / Mild / Moderate / High
Confusion or Memory Issues	None / Mild / Moderate / Severe
Agitation or Restlessness	None / Mild / Moderate / Severe
Social Interaction	Engaged / Quiet / Withdrawn
Communication Ability	Normal / Slower / Difficulty Speaking
Cooperation With Care	Cooperative / Resistant
Sleep Disturbance	Yes / No

Behaviour Changes Observed

Describe any unusual or new behaviours noticed today.

Examples: wandering, repeated questions, sudden anger, unusual quietness, confusion about time or place.

Possible Triggers

If a behavioural change occurred, note anything that may have triggered it.

Examples: loud environment, fatigue, medication change, unfamiliar surroundings.

Activities Today

Sometimes activities can affect mood or behaviour.

Activities completed today:

☐ Light exercise
☐ Conversation with family or friends
☐ Reading or puzzles
☐ Music or relaxation
☐ Outdoor time
☐ Doctor visit
☐ Other: ___________________

Notes:

Calming Strategies Used

If the person became upset, what helped calm them?

Examples: reassurance, quiet environment, music, rest.

Caregiver Notes

Record anything important you may want to discuss with a doctor or healthcare provider.

Daily Mood & Behaviour Log

Date: ______________________

Observation Category	Record / Notes
Overall Mood	Happy / Calm / Neutral / Irritable / Sad
Anxiety Level	None / Mild / Moderate / High
Confusion or Memory Issues	None / Mild / Moderate / Severe
Agitation or Restlessness	None / Mild / Moderate / Severe
Social Interaction	Engaged / Quiet / Withdrawn
Communication Ability	Normal / Slower / Difficulty Speaking
Cooperation With Care	Cooperative / Resistant
Sleep Disturbance	Yes / No

Behaviour Changes Observed

Describe any unusual or new behaviours noticed today.

Examples: wandering, repeated questions, sudden anger, unusual quietness, confusion about time or place.

Possible Triggers

If a behavioural change occurred, note anything that may have triggered it.

Examples: loud environment, fatigue, medication change, unfamiliar surroundings.

Activities Today

Sometimes activities can affect mood or behaviour

Activities completed today:

☐ Light exercise
☐ Conversation with family or friends
☐ Reading or puzzles
☐ Music or relaxation
☐ Outdoor time
☐ Doctor visit
☐ Other: ________________

Notes:

____

____

Calming Strategies Used

If the person became upset, what helped calm them?

Examples: reassurance, quiet environment, music, rest.

____

____

____

Caregiver Notes

Record anything important you may want to discuss with a doctor or healthcare provider.

____

____

____

____

Daily Mood & Behaviour Log

Date: ______________________

Observation Category	Record / Notes
Overall Mood	Happy / Calm / Neutral / Irritable / Sad
Anxiety Level	None / Mild / Moderate / High
Confusion or Memory Issues	None / Mild / Moderate / Severe
Agitation or Restlessness	None / Mild / Moderate / Severe
Social Interaction	Engaged / Quiet / Withdrawn
Communication Ability	Normal / Slower / Difficulty Speaking
Cooperation With Care	Cooperative / Resistant
Sleep Disturbance	Yes / No

Behaviour Changes Observed

Describe any unusual or new behaviours noticed today.

Examples: wandering, repeated questions, sudden anger, unusual quietness, confusion about time or place.

Possible Triggers

If a behavioural change occurred, note anything that may have triggered it.

Examples: loud environment, fatigue, medication change, unfamiliar surroundings.

Activities Today

Sometimes activities can affect mood or behaviour

Activities completed today:

☐ Light exercise
☐ Conversation with family or friends
☐ Reading or puzzles
☐ Music or relaxation
☐ Outdoor time
☐ Doctor visit
☐ Other: ___________________

Notes:

Calming Strategies Used

If the person became upset, what helped calm them?

Examples: reassurance, quiet environment, music, rest.

Caregiver Notes

Record anything important you may want to discuss with a doctor or healthcare provider.

Daily Mood & Behaviour Log

Date: ______________________

Observation Category	Record / Notes
Overall Mood	Happy / Calm / Neutral / Irritable / Sad
Anxiety Level	None / Mild / Moderate / High
Confusion or Memory Issues	None / Mild / Moderate / Severe
Agitation or Restlessness	None / Mild / Moderate / Severe
Social Interaction	Engaged / Quiet / Withdrawn
Communication Ability	Normal / Slower / Difficulty Speaking
Cooperation With Care	Cooperative / Resistant
Sleep Disturbance	Yes / No

Behaviour Changes Observed

Describe any unusual or new behaviours noticed today.

Examples: wandering, repeated questions, sudden anger, unusual quietness, confusion about time or place.

Possible Triggers

If a behavioural change occurred, note anything that may have triggered it.

Examples: loud environment, fatigue, medication change, unfamiliar surroundings.

Activities Today

Sometimes activities can affect mood or behaviour

Activities completed today:

☐ Light exercise
☐ Conversation with family or friends
☐ Reading or puzzles
☐ Music or relaxation
☐ Outdoor time
☐ Doctor visit
☐ Other: ___________________

Notes:

Calming Strategies Used

If the person became upset, what helped calm them?

Examples: reassurance, quiet environment, music, rest.

Caregiver Notes

Record anything important you may want to discuss with a doctor or healthcare provider.

Section 5
Doctor Visits & Appointment Tracker

Regular medical appointments are an important part of managing health conditions and monitoring overall well-being. During these visits, doctors may provide important updates, treatment recommendations, or medication adjustments.

However, it can sometimes be difficult to remember everything discussed during an appointment. Writing down key points helps caregivers stay organized and ensures that instructions from healthcare professionals are not forgotten.

This section is designed to help you prepare for medical visits, record important information during the appointment, and track follow-up actions afterward.

Bringing this logbook to appointments can also help doctors better understand the patient's daily health patterns.

Appointment Preparation

Before the appointment, take a few minutes to note the purpose of the visit and any questions you would like to ask the doctor.

Appointment Date: ______________________

Doctor / Specialist Name: ______________________

Clinic / Hospital: ______________________

Reason for Visit:

____

Questions to Ask the Doctor:

1. ____
2. ____
3. ____
4. ____

____

Appointment Notes

Use this section during the visit to record important information shared by the doctor.

Diagnosis or Health Update:

____

____

Tests Recommended:

____

Medication Changes:

____

Doctor's Advice or Instructions:

____

____

____

Follow-Up Actions

Next Appointment Date: ______________________

Tests or Procedures Scheduled:

____

Lifestyle or Care Recommendations:

____

Medication Changes to Monitor:

____

Additional Notes:

____

____

____

Appointment Summary Tracker

Date	Doctor	Reason for Visit	Key Outcome	Next Visit

Appointment Preparation

Before the appointment, take a few minutes to note the purpose of the visit and any questions you would like to ask the doctor.

Appointment Date: ______________________

Doctor / Specialist Name: ______________________

Clinic / Hospital: ______________________

Reason for Visit:

Questions to Ask the Doctor:

1.
2.
3.
4.

Appointment Notes

Use this section during the visit to record important information shared by the doctor.

Diagnosis or Health Update:

Tests Recommended:

Medication Changes:

Doctor's Advice or Instructions:

Follow-Up Actions

Next Appointment Date: ______________________

Tests or Procedures Scheduled:

Lifestyle or Care Recommendations:

Medication Changes to Monitor:

Additional Notes:

Appointment Summary Tracker

Date	Doctor	Reason for Visit	Key Outcome	Next Visit

Appointment Preparation

Before the appointment, take a few minutes to note the purpose of the visit and any questions you would like to ask the doctor.

Appointment Date: ______________________

Doctor / Specialist Name: ______________________

Clinic / Hospital: ______________________

Reason for Visit:

____

Questions to Ask the Doctor:

1. ____
2. ____
3. ____
4. ____

____

Appointment Notes

Use this section during the visit to record important information shared by the doctor.

Diagnosis or Health Update:

____

____

Tests Recommended:

____

Medication Changes:

____

Doctor's Advice or Instructions:

____

____

____

Follow-Up Actions

Next Appointment Date: ______________________

Tests or Procedures Scheduled:

____

Lifestyle or Care Recommendations:

____

Medication Changes to Monitor:

____

Additional Notes:

____

____

____

Appointment Summary Tracker

Date	Doctor	Reason for Visit	Key Outcome	Next Visit

Appointment Preparation

Before the appointment, take a few minutes to note the purpose of the visit and any questions you would like to ask the doctor.

Appointment Date: ______________________

Doctor / Specialist Name: ______________________

Clinic / Hospital: ______________________

Reason for Visit:

____

Questions to Ask the Doctor:

1. ____
2. ____
3. ____
4. ____

____

Appointment Notes

Use this section during the visit to record important information shared by the doctor.

Diagnosis or Health Update:

____

____

Tests Recommended:

____

Medication Changes:

____

Doctor's Advice or Instructions:

____

____

____

Follow-Up Actions

Next Appointment Date: ______________________

Tests or Procedures Scheduled:

____

Lifestyle or Care Recommendations:

____

Medication Changes to Monitor:

____

Additional Notes:

____

____

____

Appointment Summary Tracker

Date	Doctor	Reason for Visit	Key Outcome	Next Visit

Appointment Preparation

Before the appointment, take a few minutes to note the purpose of the visit and any questions you would like to ask the doctor.

Appointment Date: ______________________

Doctor / Specialist Name: ______________________

Clinic / Hospital: ______________________

Reason for Visit:

Questions to Ask the Doctor:

1. ______________________
2. ______________________
3. ______________________
4. ______________________

Appointment Notes

Use this section during the visit to record important information shared by the doctor.

Diagnosis or Health Update:

Tests Recommended:

Medication Changes:

Doctor's Advice or Instructions:

Follow-Up Actions

Next Appointment Date: ______________________

Tests or Procedures Scheduled:

Lifestyle or Care Recommendations:

Medication Changes to Monitor:

Additional Notes:

Appointment Summary Tracker

Date	Doctor	Reason for Visit	Key Outcome	Next Visit

Appointment Preparation

Before the appointment, take a few minutes to note the purpose of the visit and any questions you would like to ask the doctor.

Appointment Date: ______________________

Doctor / Specialist Name: ______________________

Clinic / Hospital: ______________________

Reason for Visit:

Questions to Ask the Doctor:

1.
2.
3.
4.

Appointment Notes

Use this section during the visit to record important information shared by the doctor.

Diagnosis or Health Update:

Tests Recommended:

Medication Changes:

Doctor's Advice or Instructions:

Follow-Up Actions

Next Appointment Date: ______________________

Tests or Procedures Scheduled:

Lifestyle or Care Recommendations:

Medication Changes to Monitor:

Additional Notes:

Appointment Summary Tracker

Date	Doctor	Reason for Visit	Key Outcome	Next Visit

Appointment Preparation

Before the appointment, take a few minutes to note the purpose of the visit and any questions you would like to ask the doctor.

Appointment Date: ______________________

Doctor / Specialist Name: ______________________

Clinic / Hospital: ______________________

Reason for Visit:

Questions to Ask the Doctor:

1.
2.
3.
4.

Appointment Notes

Use this section during the visit to record important information shared by the doctor.

Diagnosis or Health Update:

Tests Recommended:

Medication Changes:

Doctor's Advice or Instructions:

Follow-Up Actions

Next Appointment Date: ______________________

Tests or Procedures Scheduled:

Lifestyle or Care Recommendations:

Medication Changes to Monitor:

Additional Notes:

Appointment Summary Tracker

Date	Doctor	Reason for Visit	Key Outcome	Next Visit

Appointment Preparation

Before the appointment, take a few minutes to note the purpose of the visit and any questions you would like to ask the doctor.

Appointment Date: ______________________

Doctor / Specialist Name: ______________________

Clinic / Hospital: ______________________

Reason for Visit:

____

Questions to Ask the Doctor:

1. ____
2. ____
3. ____
4. ____

____

Appointment Notes

Use this section during the visit to record important information shared by the doctor.

Diagnosis or Health Update:

____

____

Tests Recommended:

____

Medication Changes:

____

Doctor's Advice or Instructions:

____

____

____

Follow-Up Actions

Next Appointment Date: ______________________

Tests or Procedures Scheduled:

Lifestyle or Care Recommendations:

Medication Changes to Monitor:

Additional Notes:

Appointment Summary Tracker

Date	Doctor	Reason for Visit	Key Outcome	Next Visit

Appointment Preparation

Before the appointment, take a few minutes to note the purpose of the visit and any questions you would like to ask the doctor.

Appointment Date: ______________________

Doctor / Specialist Name: ______________________

Clinic / Hospital: ______________________

Reason for Visit:

____

Questions to Ask the Doctor:

1. ____
2. ____
3. ____
4. ____

____

Appointment Notes

Use this section during the visit to record important information shared by the doctor.

Diagnosis or Health Update:

____

____

Tests Recommended:

____

Medication Changes:

____

Doctor's Advice or Instructions:

____

____

____

Follow-Up Actions

Next Appointment Date: ______________________

Tests or Procedures Scheduled:

____

Lifestyle or Care Recommendations:

____

Medication Changes to Monitor:

____

Additional Notes:

____

____

____

Appointment Summary Tracker

Date	Doctor	Reason for Visit	Key Outcome	Next Visit

Appointment Preparation

Before the appointment, take a few minutes to note the purpose of the visit and any questions you would like to ask the doctor.

Appointment Date: ______________________

Doctor / Specialist Name: ______________________

Clinic / Hospital: ______________________

Reason for Visit:

____

Questions to Ask the Doctor:

1. ____
2. ____
3. ____
4. ____

____

Appointment Notes

Use this section during the visit to record important information shared by the doctor.

Diagnosis or Health Update:

____

____

Tests Recommended:

____

Medication Changes:

____

Doctor's Advice or Instructions:

____

____

____

Follow-Up Actions

Next Appointment Date: ______________________

Tests or Procedures Scheduled:

____

Lifestyle or Care Recommendations:

____

Medication Changes to Monitor:

____

Additional Notes:

____

____

____

Appointment Summary Tracker

Date	Doctor	Reason for Visit	Key Outcome	Next Visit

Appointment Preparation

Before the appointment, take a few minutes to note the purpose of the visit and any questions you would like to ask the doctor.

Appointment Date: ______________________

Doctor / Specialist Name: ______________________

Clinic / Hospital: ______________________

Reason for Visit:

____

Questions to Ask the Doctor:

1. ____
2. ____
3. ____
4. ____

____

Appointment Notes

Use this section during the visit to record important information shared by the doctor.

Diagnosis or Health Update:

____

____

Tests Recommended:

____

Medication Changes:

____

Doctor's Advice or Instructions:

____

____

____

Follow-Up Actions

Next Appointment Date: ______________________

Tests or Procedures Scheduled:

____

Lifestyle or Care Recommendations:

____

Medication Changes to Monitor:

____

Additional Notes:

____

____

____

Appointment Summary Tracker

Date	Doctor	Reason for Visit	Key Outcome	Next Visit

Appointment Preparation

Before the appointment, take a few minutes to note the purpose of the visit and any questions you would like to ask the doctor.

Appointment Date: ______________________

Doctor / Specialist Name: ______________________

Clinic / Hospital: ______________________

Reason for Visit:

Questions to Ask the Doctor:

1.
2.
3.
4.

Appointment Notes

Use this section during the visit to record important information shared by the doctor.

Diagnosis or Health Update:

Tests Recommended:

Medication Changes:

Doctor's Advice or Instructions:

Follow-Up Actions

Next Appointment Date: ______________________

Tests or Procedures Scheduled:

____

Lifestyle or Care Recommendations:

____

Medication Changes to Monitor:

____

Additional Notes:

____

____

____

Appointment Summary Tracker

Date	Doctor	Reason for Visit	Key Outcome	Next Visit

Appointment Preparation

Before the appointment, take a few minutes to note the purpose of the visit and any questions you would like to ask the doctor.

Appointment Date: ______________________

Doctor / Specialist Name: ______________________

Clinic / Hospital: ______________________

Reason for Visit:

____

Questions to Ask the Doctor:

1. ____
2. ____
3. ____
4. ____

____

Appointment Notes

Use this section during the visit to record important information shared by the doctor.

Diagnosis or Health Update:

____

____

Tests Recommended:

____

Medication Changes:

____

Doctor's Advice or Instructions:

____

____

____

Follow-Up Actions

Next Appointment Date: ______________________

Tests or Procedures Scheduled:

____

Lifestyle or Care Recommendations:

____

Medication Changes to Monitor:

____

Additional Notes:

____

____

____

Appointment Summary Tracker

Date	**Doctor**	**Reason for Visit**	**Key Outcome**	**Next Visit**

Appointment Preparation

Before the appointment, take a few minutes to note the purpose of the visit and any questions you would like to ask the doctor.

Appointment Date: ______________________

Doctor / Specialist Name: ______________________

Clinic / Hospital: ______________________

Reason for Visit:

____

Questions to Ask the Doctor:

1. ____
2. ____
3. ____
4. ____

____

Appointment Notes

Use this section during the visit to record important information shared by the doctor.

Diagnosis or Health Update:

____

____

Tests Recommended:

____

Medication Changes:

____

Doctor's Advice or Instructions:

____

____

____

Follow-Up Actions

Next Appointment Date: ______________________

Tests or Procedures Scheduled:

Lifestyle or Care Recommendations:

Medication Changes to Monitor:

Additional Notes:

Appointment Summary Tracker

Date	Doctor	Reason for Visit	Key Outcome	Next Visit

Appointment Preparation

Before the appointment, take a few minutes to note the purpose of the visit and any questions you would like to ask the doctor.

Appointment Date: ______________________

Doctor / Specialist Name: ______________________

Clinic / Hospital: ______________________

Reason for Visit:

Questions to Ask the Doctor:

1.
2.
3.
4.

Appointment Notes

Use this section during the visit to record important information shared by the doctor.

Diagnosis or Health Update:

Tests Recommended:

Medication Changes:

Doctor's Advice or Instructions:

Follow-Up Actions

Next Appointment Date: ______________________

Tests or Procedures Scheduled:

Lifestyle or Care Recommendations:

Medication Changes to Monitor:

Additional Notes:

Appointment Summary Tracker

Date	Doctor	Reason for Visit	Key Outcome	Next Visit

Section 6
Caregiver Reflection & Self-Care

Caring for another person is an act of compassion, patience, and dedication. While caregivers focus most of their attention on the person they support, it is also important to remember that caregivers need care too.

Many caregivers experience physical exhaustion, emotional stress, and moments of uncertainty. Taking a few minutes to reflect on your own well-being can help you stay balanced, prevent burnout, and continue providing the best care possible.

This section is designed to give caregivers a quiet space to pause, reflect, and acknowledge their own experiences. Writing down thoughts, feelings, and observations can be helpful for maintaining emotional strength and perspective.

There is no right or wrong way to use these pages. Simply write honestly about your experiences and how you are feeling.

Remember: taking care of yourself is not selfish — it is an important part of being a strong and sustainable caregiver.

Weekly Caregiver Reflection

Week 1 Week Starting: ______________________

How was the overall health of the person I am caring for this week?

What positive moments did I notice this week?

What challenges did I experience this week?

What concerns should I discuss with a doctor or healthcare professional?

My Well-Being This Week

How would I describe my stress level this week?

☐ Very Low
☐ Manageable
☐ Moderate
☐ High
☐ Very High

What emotions did I experience most this week?

☐ Calm
☐ Hopeful
☐ Tired
☐ Frustrated
☐ Overwhelmed
☐ Grateful
☐ Other: ______________________

Notes:

Self-Care Check-In

Did I take time for myself this week?

☐ Yes
☐ A little
☐ Not really

Things that helped me relax or recharge:

☐ Walking or exercise
☐ Talking with friends or family
☐ Reading or music
☐ Quiet rest or meditation
☐ Personal hobbies
☐ Other: ______________________

What is one small thing I can do next week for my own well-being?

____

____

Gratitude Reflection

Even during difficult times, small moments of gratitude can help maintain emotional balance.

This week I am grateful for:

1. ______________________________________
2. ______________________________________
3. ______________________________________

Personal Notes

Use this space to write any thoughts, experiences, or reflections about your caregiving journey.

____

____

____

____

Weekly Caregiver Reflection

Week 2 Week Starting: ______________________

How was the overall health of the person I am caring for this week?

What positive moments did I notice this week?

What challenges did I experience this week?

What concerns should I discuss with a doctor or healthcare professional?

My Well-Being This Week

How would I describe my stress level this week?

☐ Very Low
☐ Manageable
☐ Moderate
☐ High
☐ Very High

What emotions did I experience most this week?

☐ Calm
☐ Hopeful
☐ Tired
☐ Frustrated
☐ Overwhelmed
☐ Grateful
☐ Other: ______________________

Notes:

Self-Care Check-In

Did I take time for myself this week?

☐ Yes
☐ A little
☐ Not really

Things that helped me relax or recharge:

☐ Walking or exercise
☐ Talking with friends or family
☐ Reading or music
☐ Quiet rest or meditation
☐ Personal hobbies
☐ Other: ______________________

What is one small thing I can do next week for my own well-being?

____

____

Gratitude Reflection

Even during difficult times, small moments of gratitude can help maintain emotional balance.

This week I am grateful for:

1. ____
2. ____
3. ____

Personal Notes

Use this space to write any thoughts, experiences, or reflections about your caregiving journey.

____

____

____

____

Weekly Caregiver Reflection

Week 3 Week Starting: ______________________

How was the overall health of the person I am caring for this week?

What positive moments did I notice this week?

What challenges did I experience this week?

What concerns should I discuss with a doctor or healthcare professional?

My Well-Being This Week

How would I describe my stress level this week?

☐ Very Low
☐ Manageable
☐ Moderate
☐ High
☐ Very High

What emotions did I experience most this week?

☐ Calm
☐ Hopeful
☐ Tired
☐ Frustrated
☐ Overwhelmed
☐ Grateful
☐ Other: ______________________

Notes:

Self-Care Check-In

Did I take time for myself this week?

☐ Yes
☐ A little
☐ Not really

Things that helped me relax or recharge:

☐ Walking or exercise
☐ Talking with friends or family
☐ Reading or music
☐ Quiet rest or meditation
☐ Personal hobbies
☐ Other: ______________________

What is one small thing I can do next week for my own well-being?

____

____

Gratitude Reflection

Even during difficult times, small moments of gratitude can help maintain emotional balance.

This week I am grateful for:

1. ____
2. ____
3. ____

Personal Notes

Use this space to write any thoughts, experiences, or reflections about your caregiving journey.

____

____

____

____

Weekly Caregiver Reflection

Week 4 Week Starting: ______________________

How was the overall health of the person I am caring for this week?

What positive moments did I notice this week?

What challenges did I experience this week?

What concerns should I discuss with a doctor or healthcare professional?

My Well-Being This Week

How would I describe my stress level this week?

☐ Very Low
☐ Manageable
☐ Moderate
☐ High
☐ Very High

What emotions did I experience most this week?

☐ Calm
☐ Hopeful
☐ Tired
☐ Frustrated
☐ Overwhelmed
☐ Grateful
☐ Other: ______________________

Notes:

Self-Care Check-In

Did I take time for myself this week?

☐ Yes
☐ A little
☐ Not really

Things that helped me relax or recharge:

☐ Walking or exercise
☐ Talking with friends or family
☐ Reading or music
☐ Quiet rest or meditation
☐ Personal hobbies
☐ Other: ______________________

What is one small thing I can do next week for my own well-being?

____

____

Gratitude Reflection

Even during difficult times, small moments of gratitude can help maintain emotional balance.

This week I am grateful for:

1. ____
2. ____
3. ____

Personal Notes

Use this space to write any thoughts, experiences, or reflections about your caregiving journey.

____

____

____

____

Weekly Caregiver Reflection

Week 5 Week Starting: ______________________

How was the overall health of the person I am caring for this week?

What positive moments did I notice this week?

What challenges did I experience this week?

What concerns should I discuss with a doctor or healthcare professional?

My Well-Being This Week

How would I describe my stress level this week?

- ☐ Very Low
- ☐ Manageable
- ☐ Moderate
- ☐ High
- ☐ Very High

What emotions did I experience most this week?

- ☐ Calm
- ☐ Hopeful
- ☐ Tired
- ☐ Frustrated
- ☐ Overwhelmed
- ☐ Grateful
- ☐ Other: ______________________

Notes:

Self-Care Check-In

Did I take time for myself this week?

☐ Yes
☐ A little
☐ Not really

Things that helped me relax or recharge:

☐ Walking or exercise
☐ Talking with friends or family
☐ Reading or music
☐ Quiet rest or meditation
☐ Personal hobbies
☐ Other: ______________________

What is one small thing I can do next week for my own well-being?

____

____

Gratitude Reflection

Even during difficult times, small moments of gratitude can help maintain emotional balance.

This week I am grateful for:

1. ______________________________________
2. ______________________________________
3. ______________________________________

Personal Notes

Use this space to write any thoughts, experiences, or reflections about your caregiving journey.

____

____

____

____

Weekly Caregiver Reflection

Week 6 Week Starting: ______________________

How was the overall health of the person I am caring for this week?

What positive moments did I notice this week?

What challenges did I experience this week?

What concerns should I discuss with a doctor or healthcare professional?

My Well-Being This Week

How would I describe my stress level this week?

☐ Very Low
☐ Manageable
☐ Moderate
☐ High
☐ Very High

What emotions did I experience most this week?

☐ Calm
☐ Hopeful
☐ Tired
☐ Frustrated
☐ Overwhelmed
☐ Grateful
☐ Other: ______________________

Notes:

Self-Care Check-In

Did I take time for myself this week?

☐ Yes
☐ A little
☐ Not really

Things that helped me relax or recharge:

☐ Walking or exercise
☐ Talking with friends or family
☐ Reading or music
☐ Quiet rest or meditation
☐ Personal hobbies
☐ Other: ______________________

What is one small thing I can do next week for my own well-being?

____

____

Gratitude Reflection

Even during difficult times, small moments of gratitude can help maintain emotional balance.

This week I am grateful for:

1. ____
2. ____
3. ____

Personal Notes

Use this space to write any thoughts, experiences, or reflections about your caregiving journey.

____

____

____

____

Weekly Caregiver Reflection

Week 7 Week Starting: ______________________

How was the overall health of the person I am caring for this week?

What positive moments did I notice this week?

What challenges did I experience this week?

What concerns should I discuss with a doctor or healthcare professional?

My Well-Being This Week

How would I describe my stress level this week?

☐ Very Low

☐ Manageable

☐ Moderate

☐ High

☐ Very High

What emotions did I experience most this week?

☐ Calm

☐ Hopeful

☐ Tired

☐ Frustrated

☐ Overwhelmed

☐ Grateful

☐ Other: ______________________

Notes:

Self-Care Check-In

Did I take time for myself this week?

☐ Yes
☐ A little
☐ Not really

Things that helped me relax or recharge:

☐ Walking or exercise
☐ Talking with friends or family
☐ Reading or music
☐ Quiet rest or meditation
☐ Personal hobbies
☐ Other: ______________________

What is one small thing I can do next week for my own well-being?

____

____

Gratitude Reflection

Even during difficult times, small moments of gratitude can help maintain emotional balance.

This week I am grateful for:

1. ____
2. ____
3. ____

Personal Notes

Use this space to write any thoughts, experiences, or reflections about your caregiving journey.

____

____

____

____

Weekly Caregiver Reflection

Week 8 Week Starting: ______________________

How was the overall health of the person I am caring for this week?

What positive moments did I notice this week?

What challenges did I experience this week?

What concerns should I discuss with a doctor or healthcare professional?

My Well-Being This Week

How would I describe my stress level this week?

☐ Very Low

☐ Manageable

☐ Moderate

☐ High

☐ Very High

What emotions did I experience most this week?

☐ Calm

☐ Hopeful

☐ Tired

☐ Frustrated

☐ Overwhelmed

☐ Grateful

☐ Other: ______________________

Notes:

Self-Care Check-In

Did I take time for myself this week?

☐ Yes
☐ A little
☐ Not really

Things that helped me relax or recharge:

☐ Walking or exercise
☐ Talking with friends or family
☐ Reading or music
☐ Quiet rest or meditation
☐ Personal hobbies
☐ Other: ______________________

What is one small thing I can do next week for my own well-being?

____

____

Gratitude Reflection

Even during difficult times, small moments of gratitude can help maintain emotional balance.

This week I am grateful for:

1. ____
2. ____
3. ____

Personal Notes

Use this space to write any thoughts, experiences, or reflections about your caregiving journey.

____

____

____

____

Weekly Caregiver Reflection

Week 9 Week Starting: ______________________

How was the overall health of the person I am caring for this week?

What positive moments did I notice this week?

What challenges did I experience this week?

What concerns should I discuss with a doctor or healthcare professional?

My Well-Being This Week

How would I describe my stress level this week?

☐ Very Low
☐ Manageable
☐ Moderate
☐ High
☐ Very High

What emotions did I experience most this week?

☐ Calm
☐ Hopeful
☐ Tired
☐ Frustrated
☐ Overwhelmed
☐ Grateful
☐ Other: ______________________

Notes:

Self-Care Check-In

Did I take time for myself this week?

☐ Yes
☐ A little
☐ Not really

Things that helped me relax or recharge:

☐ Walking or exercise
☐ Talking with friends or family
☐ Reading or music
☐ Quiet rest or meditation
☐ Personal hobbies
☐ Other: ______________________

What is one small thing I can do next week for my own well-being?

____

____

Gratitude Reflection

Even during difficult times, small moments of gratitude can help maintain emotional balance.

This week I am grateful for:

1. ____
2. ____
3. ____

Personal Notes

Use this space to write any thoughts, experiences, or reflections about your caregiving journey.

____

____

____

____

Weekly Caregiver Reflection

Week 10 Week Starting: ______________________

How was the overall health of the person I am caring for this week?

What positive moments did I notice this week?

What challenges did I experience this week?

What concerns should I discuss with a doctor or healthcare professional?

My Well-Being This Week

How would I describe my stress level this week?

☐ Very Low
☐ Manageable
☐ Moderate
☐ High
☐ Very High

What emotions did I experience most this week?

☐ Calm
☐ Hopeful
☐ Tired
☐ Frustrated
☐ Overwhelmed
☐ Grateful
☐ Other: ______________________

Notes:

Self-Care Check-In

Did I take time for myself this week?

☐ Yes
☐ A little
☐ Not really

Things that helped me relax or recharge:

☐ Walking or exercise
☐ Talking with friends or family
☐ Reading or music
☐ Quiet rest or meditation
☐ Personal hobbies
☐ Other: ______________________

What is one small thing I can do next week for my own well-being?

____

____

Gratitude Reflection

Even during difficult times, small moments of gratitude can help maintain emotional balance.

This week I am grateful for:

1. ____
2. ____
3. ____

Personal Notes

Use this space to write any thoughts, experiences, or reflections about your caregiving journey.

____

____

____

____

Weekly Caregiver Reflection

Week 11 Week Starting: ______________________

How was the overall health of the person I am caring for this week?

____

What positive moments did I notice this week?

____

What challenges did I experience this week?

____

What concerns should I discuss with a doctor or healthcare professional?

____

____

My Well-Being This Week

How would I describe my stress level this week?

☐ Very Low
☐ Manageable
☐ Moderate
☐ High
☐ Very High

What emotions did I experience most this week?

☐ Calm
☐ Hopeful
☐ Tired
☐ Frustrated
☐ Overwhelmed
☐ Grateful
☐ Other: ______________________

Notes:

____

Self-Care Check-In

Did I take time for myself this week?

☐ Yes

☐ A little

☐ Not really

Things that helped me relax or recharge:

☐ Walking or exercise

☐ Talking with friends or family

☐ Reading or music

☐ Quiet rest or meditation

☐ Personal hobbies

☐ Other: ______________________

What is one small thing I can do next week for my own well-being?

____

____

Gratitude Reflection

Even during difficult times, small moments of gratitude can help maintain emotional balance.

This week I am grateful for:

1. ______________________________________
2. ______________________________________
3. ______________________________________

Personal Notes

Use this space to write any thoughts, experiences, or reflections about your caregiving journey.

____

____

____

____

Weekly Caregiver Reflection

Week 12 Week Starting: ______________________

How was the overall health of the person I am caring for this week?

What positive moments did I notice this week?

What challenges did I experience this week?

What concerns should I discuss with a doctor or healthcare professional?

My Well-Being This Week

How would I describe my stress level this week?

☐ Very Low
☐ Manageable
☐ Moderate
☐ High
☐ Very High

What emotions did I experience most this week?

☐ Calm
☐ Hopeful
☐ Tired
☐ Frustrated
☐ Overwhelmed
☐ Grateful
☐ Other: ______________________

Notes:

Self-Care Check-In

Did I take time for myself this week?

☐ Yes
☐ A little
☐ Not really

Things that helped me relax or recharge:

☐ Walking or exercise
☐ Talking with friends or family
☐ Reading or music
☐ Quiet rest or meditation
☐ Personal hobbies
☐ Other: ______________________

What is one small thing I can do next week for my own well-being?

____

____

Gratitude Reflection

Even during difficult times, small moments of gratitude can help maintain emotional balance.

This week I am grateful for:

1. ______________________________________
2. ______________________________________
3. ______________________________________

Personal Notes

Use this space to write any thoughts, experiences, or reflections about your caregiving journey.

____

____

____

____

A Final Note for Caregivers

Caregiving is one of the most meaningful and selfless roles a person can take on.

Every day you offer your time, patience, and compassion to someone who needs support. Many of the things you do may seem small in the moment — helping with medication, preparing meals, offering reassurance, or simply being present — but these acts of care make an enormous difference.

Caregiving can also be challenging.

There may be days when you feel tired, uncertain, or overwhelmed. Those feelings are completely natural. Caring for another person requires emotional strength, and it is important to recognize the effort you put in each day.

Remember that you are not alone on this journey.

Healthcare professionals, family members, friends, and support communities can all play a role in helping caregivers manage responsibilities and maintain their own well-being.

It is also important to remember something many caregivers forget:

Taking care of yourself is part of taking care of others.

Rest when you can.
Ask for help when you need it.
Celebrate small improvements and meaningful moments.

Caregiving is not about being perfect. It is about showing compassion, patience, and kindness through everyday actions.

The notes and records you have kept in this logbook may help doctors provide better care, but they also tell the story of your dedication and commitment.

And that dedication matters more than you may realize.

Thank you for the care you give, the strength you show, and the difference you make every day.

www.ingramcontent.com/pod-product-compliance
Lightning Source LLC
LaVergne TN
LVHW080038210926
848481LV00011B/3222
9798233446382